About the Author

Kathryn Marsden is well-known as the author of the best-selling *Food Combining Diet*, *Food Combining in 30 Days*, *The Food Combiner's Meal Planner*, and *Kathryn Marsden's Super Skin*. Her titles are now famous around the world and have been translated into a number of languages including Chinese, Dutch, Finnish, Bulgarian, Czech and Hebrew.

A welcome guest on both radio and TV, Kathryn has contributed to many different television programmes in the UK, Ireland, Australia and the Far East, both on-screen and behind the scenes, and is presenter of the bestselling food combining fitness video, *The One to One Option*.

Kathryn has her own health and beauty helpline with the BBC in the South-West of England and enjoys regular visits to other BBC and independent radio stations nationwide. Dynamic and enthusiastic, her warm and friendly personality, and exceptional knowledge in her chosen field are welcomed by producers, presenters and editors the world over. During the past six years, her feature articles have appeared regularly in most of the mainstream women's magazines and health press including *Cosmopolitan*, *Company Magazine*, *New Woman*, *Woman's Weekly*, and *Zest*. Kathryn is a Member of the Guild of Health Writers.

More recently, Kathryn has carved a niche in the international seminar circuit giving accredited lectures in herapeutics to practitioners of both complementary and orthodox medicine. Notable for her lighthearted presentations, she shares her knowledge of safe and effective weight loss, her sideways view of silly diets and her commonsense tips on how to survive and thrive in a frantic world. Her most recent tour of Australia, Singapore and Malaysia was a sell-out.

As far as other interests are concerned, she readily admits to being 'cat crazy, gardening mad, a Classic FM junkie and happily married, not necessarily in that order'.

Kathryn's nutrition studies began as a direct result of her husband Ralph being diagnosed with cancer in 1984. Although he was only given a few weeks to live, Ralph is now celebrating his eleventh year of recovery.

Also by Kathryn Marsden

Food Combining Diet
Food Combining In 30 Days
The Food Combiner's Meal Planner
Kathryn Marsden's Super Skin

ALL DAY ENERGY

The Stress-Free Way to Revitalize Your Health

Kathryn Marsden

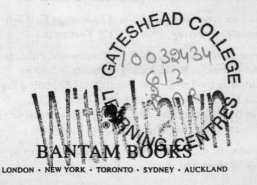

BANTAM BOOKS

LONDON · NEW YORK · TORONTO · SYDNEY · AUCKLAND

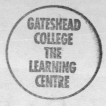

ALL DAY ENERGY
A BANTAM BOOK: 0 553 40849 6

First Publication in Great Britain

PRINTING HISTORY
Bantam edition published 1995

Set in Linotype Garamond 3 and Monotype Gill Sans by
Phoenix Typesetting, Ilkley, West Yorkshire.

Bantam Books are published by Transworld Publishers Ltd,
61–63 Uxbridge Road, Ealing, London W5 5SA,
in Australia by Transworld Publishers (Australia) Pty Ltd,
15–25 Helles Avenue, Moorebank, NSW 2170,
and in New Zealand by Transworld Publishers (NZ) Ltd,
3 William Pickering Drive, Albany, Auckland.

Reproduced, printed and bound in Great Britain by
Cox & Wyman Ltd, Reading, Berks.

This book is dedicated to Hazel and Stuart Sapcote

May those who love us, love us
And those that don't love us
May God turn their hearts;
And if He doesn't turn their hearts
May He turn their ankles
So we'll know them by their limping

Irish Proverb

Acknowledgements

My admiration, appreciation and grateful thanks go to all the talented practitioners, colleagues and friends who have helped, in so many different ways, with the preparation of this book.

***   Dr Christine Page MB, BS, MRCGP, DCH, DRCOG, MFHom. for the assistance she has given with the checking of technical and medical information in this manuscript.

***   Yoga expert, Mary Harris for her assistance with the yoga and breathing exercises.

***   Fitness teacher, Jan Robinson for the very welcome input on exercise.

***   Aromatherapist, Maggie Fillingham for the advice on aromatherapy and essential oils.

***   Eve Cameron, Francis Leinster, Tony Mulliken, Gillian Hamer and Elizabeth Ann Runyard for taking the time to read sections of the raw manuscript and for their valuable comments. Extra special thanks to Dr Tony Pickup.

***   Blackmores (UK and Sydney, Australia) for their assistance with research.

***   Bent Henriksen of Pharma Nord UK for providing so much helpful research material.

Contents

Foreword
by the Rt Hon. The Earl of Suffolk and Berkshire

I consider my chance meeting on Tuesday, 8 June 1993, with Kathryn Marsden's husband Ralph an important and special day in my life since it led to my being introduced to Kathryn. By following her recommendations (including her excellent and easy to follow advice on food combining), I am free of indigestion, am far more discriminating about my food choices *and* I feel so much better! To have the opportunity to write the Foreword to *All Day Energy* is therefore a singular honour for the pupil of the Master – or should I say 'Mistress'.

Is there anyone who would not welcome more energy? Weariness, worry and general tiredness seem to be the bane of so many people's lives but are burdens which we appear to accept as part of the daily round. In my experience, however, the limited advice thus far available has consisted mostly of the 'do this', 'don't do that' variety, issued with very little appreciation of how difficult it can be to fit such 'instructions' into an already stressed and overworked lifestyle.

All Day Energy takes a refreshingly different approach and I am impressed with the friendly and practical easy to use style of the book. Kathryn's humour and empathy reach out to the reader and she writes with knowledge and understanding on the problems of lethargy, exhaustion, chronic fatigue, weight difficulties, disturbed sleep, jet lag, workaholism and stress. Other fascinating chapters explain how the colours we choose can affect our energy, why pollution makes us tired and why certain foods can sap our stamina and affect our mood. Most importantly, Kathryn gives us realistic and effective solutions.

All Day Energy was great fun to read and I have enjoyed it thoroughly. I feel sure that you, too, will gain great benefit from its content.

Preface

Let's face it, the number of people who possess exciting, exulting energy is definitely on the slide. Tired feet drag addled brains and leaded limbs from one debilitating day to the next with no time for rest or respite. Nearly everyone you know is knackered and, whether or not they can come up with any justifiable explanations for feeling so utterly exhausted, most folks regard fatigue as a permanent and unfixable fixture in their lives. Worse still, only a few seem happy to admit that their constant state of tiredness is a problem in the first place. The ancient art of 'shimpling' (roughly translated means lying about the state of your life to cheer up your parents) is obviously alive and well. Not a good idea to make too much of a fuss. Put a brave face on it, that's the answer.

Just out of interest, how many humans can you think of who look and feel completely hunky-dory? Could it be that wide awake, full of energy people are becoming an endangered species?

Possibly, probably.

Feelings of weariness, being frayed at the edges or generally 'under par' are so common as to have become almost expectable. In a way, it would be easier to accept and understand this kind of tiredness if it were associated only with overwork; almost everyone gets tired if their workload is too heavy to allow for proper rest. But no. Today's common lethargy and lassitude is ever-present and everywhere.

House mothers, college students, supermarket shelf-stackers, office workers, child minders, high flying business executives – whether you go out each day or work in the home, unexplained fatigue can get you. From jet lag to tractor lag, it's no respecter of gender, status, income, colour or creed.

Exhaustion has become ubiquitous but, because it isn't imminently life-threatening, no-one takes it seriously. Not seriously enough, perhaps? For some, admitting to exhaustion is admitting defeat – and that would never do, would it? For others, suffering in silence may seem their only option.

Most of us, male or female, crawl out of bed completely shattered at one end of the day and/or crawl back into it at the other end of the day with no real sense of what happened to the time in between. Certainly no sense of enjoyment, elation, of feeling full of bounce or beans – or energetic good health. No time to stop and stare, talk to someone, have a cuddle. Too many genuine headaches for a genuine sex life.

'Life is one long process of getting tired.' So wrote the satirist and novelist Samuel Butler as long ago as eighteen hundred and something or other. (*Samuel Butler* 1835–1902).

Yup! Seems to be a pretty accurate description of the average you and me. But what kind of tiredness did Samuel mean? Surely not the bleary-eyed, clapped out, sapped out, everyday *living* kind of tiredness which has become so common that we almost expect it, take it for granted.

I know some people who are so persistently weary and worn that 'living' is the last thing they are doing. Coping, managing after a fashion, existing perhaps, surviving possibly – but living? Never!

Sounds like you, does it?

You're only a bit tired, I hear you say; nothing as bad as all that. You're not a workaholic or anything. There's no *obvious* reason why you're so exhausted – which is one of the reasons why you think it churlish to complain. How can you describe an indescribable kind of lethargy, anyway? You just feel kind of under par, overstretched, misunderstood; just, well . . . not so well. It'll pass.

Oh, really?

When was the last time you felt properly, absolutely, wide awake fit? A hundred and one per cent tip top, bright eyed and ready for anything at any time of day – or night? When was the last time you *didn't feel* like falling asleep mid-afternoon?

Go on, admit it. You could do with a year off from the housework, the cooking, the pressure at the office – or, at least, a week's undisturbed sleep. Well, a couple of days, anyway. But is that going to answer the problem?

Don't tell me, you're too tired to sleep.

Well, a change of routine, then. Take a break.

You can't?

No time.

Can't afford it.

Too much to do.

And what's the point? You're not exactly *ill* – exactly. Once you're hitched to the harness (vacuum cleaner, baby buggy, word processor, driver's seat), complete with nosebag to save stopping for meals, it's go, go, go until that nasty little terror called Tiredness comes back to bother you again. But you still have to keep go, go, going.

You're not the only one who feels as if they could – oh so easily – crash out on the bed you are in the process of making.

And those of you at the office . . . I bet you think the boardroom table looks like a nice place to lie down and have a nap.

Zzzzzzzzzzz . . . Quiet please.

Someone once told me that this all-too-familiar scenario is called Flapnott syndrome. Quite the opposite of what you would expect it to mean, the letters apparently stand for 'Feeling Like A Permanent Night On The Tiles'. A good description for the average human with average responsibilities, I'd say. Nearly everyone I talked to whilst researching this book admitted that they either slept badly, had difficulty sleeping, often felt as though they had been awake all night or were still exhausted after what should have been a good night's rest.

So is there anything you can do to improve things? To feel better? To rediscover your lost energy? And is there any point?

You betcha!

But first of all, it's important to try to tie down why you are tired in the first place.

That's what *All Day Energy* is all about; working out why you are tired all the time and then helping you to change things, to buck the trend, upgrading your health from foggy and foul to fine and dandy.

Have *you* ever stopped to wonder why you feel so whacked? Just part of life's rich pageant? Not enough hours in the day? Something you have to put up with? NO, NO and NO!

Do you want the good news or the good news? Well, the first good news is that there are reasons for this epidemic of modern dead beat, dead on your feet, dog-tiredness. The even greater news is that it isn't inevitable. If words such as 'refreshed', 'rested' and 'rejuvenated' are music to your enervated ears, then stay tuned.

All Day Energy is an easy-going, feel better, take-a-break kind of book which gives you practical and realistic solutions. It's also about helping to improve your long-term health, balancing your weight and putting back the 'do' in your do-wa-wa!

You weren't born tired. Young children don't get tired like adults do. Kids fall asleep at the drop of a disposable diaper – and often at the most inconvenient of moments. Frequently, they wake up at inconsiderate times too – and can be a pain in the proverbial when you're trying to pile up your own share of zeds or zees – but what the little people don't do is go around thinking, feeling or saying how worn out they are or behaving as zonked out zombies.

So what happens to change things? Why do so many of us run out of steam at about the same time we grow into pantihose or long trousers? And has it always been that way? Isn't this dogged and indefatigable fatigue a relatively recent phenomenon?

Before we'd ever heard of sick building syndrome, food additives, twenty-four hour television or plastic packaging, before anyone uttered the word 'stress', when physical exertion and fresh air were the norm, people got tired, sure – but were not often eclipsed by incurable exhaustion.

Exhaustion can be a physical, mental or an emotional problem. It can be caused by a great many different things from overwork and ill health through to diet, lifestyle and environment. Worst of all, it can be lonely. It can make you want to cry with frustration because you wish you felt much less tired and wonder if you ever will feel full of life again. It can make you feel guilty about feeling guilty ('but my family needs me . . .')

Good one that.

How much use do you think you'll be to your family when you've driven yourself so far down the road to complete exhaustion that you are piled up in a hospital bed, a wheelchair or dead?

How do I know all this? Well, I've been there, seen it, suffered it, felt sorry for myself, sorted it and survived.

My energy lows were brought on by an accumulation of occurrences. Trying to keep a full-time job going, being the only breadwinner of the family, nursing a sick relative, running the home, doing the weekly shopping, etc., etc. (lots of etceteras); all at once and all adding up to a serious case of overwork, over-stress and about as under-par as it is possible to be. I can reveal that eating and sleeping were way down at the bottom of my list of priorities. In the middle of this jumble – and many years before my first book was published – I was also trying to break into magazine writing. Insanity in the family, probably.

During school, writing was my first love. No, sorry, my *original* first love was a boy in the sixth form whom I adored, hopelessly and painfully, from the age of eleven. But even in my most depressed and lovesick moments, I could always find the wherewithal for a story – usually a silly one, probably to hide my abject misery that the Greek god in grey didn't even know I existed. And I wasn't all that bad at writing. Terrible at everything else but – essays and prose of sorts – untouchable. I hit the big time at age thirteen when I found my poems were welcomed by the local newspaper.

In my exhausted state, years later, I should have known better than to squeeze out what little bit of energy I had left and try to get an appointment with one of the grand women's magazines in London.

'Who did you say you were?' was the first question asked by the editor's assistant's assistant secretary when I was eventually connected.

'Kathryn Marsden.'

'Who?'

'K-a-t-h-r-y-n M-a-r-s-d-e-n.'

'*Who?*'

'Joan Collins.'

'What is it about, Joan?' (Just proves they don't listen.)

'It's about an article which I submitted to Ms . . .'

'She's gone for her sun bed,' said the monotone voice.

'*She's gone to buy a sun bed?*'

'She's gone to top up her tan, dear.'

(Roughly translated, 'dear' means 'why is this low life country bumpkin bothering me?')

'Anyway, I know we don't take work from people who have no experience' (now why did she assume that I had no experience?).

'I do have experience,' I began.

(What I want to know is, how does a person ever get experience if no-one ever gives a person a chance to get experience?)

'Hold on, I'll see.' Bored sounding sigh; 'please' would have been nice.

While holding, for a-g-e-s, I heard the same voice groaning to a colleague 'Why does anyone who has ever written a composition at school think they have the talent to write features for us? Probably couldn't come up with more than 250 words tops.'

(I swear this really happened.)

I put down the phone and burst into tears. My exhaustion was complete. I collapsed, literally. The doctor was called and I was ordered to bed, no excuses allowed. To this day, I think I may owe him my life.

Please, please don't ever get that tired.

When I recovered, I did begin writing for magazines and since then, have written features for most of them. I'll always be grateful to the health and beauty editors who gave me my early breaks and I thank them for listening and encouraging me. In particular, Chrissie Painell, Eve Cameron at *Zest*, Susan Wilson at *Cosmopolitan*, Tara Barker at *Company* and Francis Quinn at *Woman's Weekly*. Something wicked inside me still wishes I had written down the name of the arrogant monotone twerp at Pompous & Presumptuous Publishing Plc. But, of course, she wouldn't know I eventually made a career out of writing, with books in the bestseller lists. Even if she remembered my call, which I very much doubt, she still thinks my name is Joan.

It took me a long time to learn the lesson.

The one which asks 'What is it going to matter in a hundred years' time?' The one which said it was OK to say 'No' to extra work every now and then. The one which taught me that I could achieve just as much in a day as I always have done but without feeling wretched, resentful and drained, but that if I didn't, there was no need to feel guilty about it. The world won't suddenly stop turning.

A radical change for someone who had always been a slave to the saying that anything worth doing was worth doing frenetically. My mother once asked me if I used a spirit level when I put the ironing away into the airing cupboard. How can I help it if I like the towels and sheets in straight lines? Good job poor old Freud has been debunked. He'd have had a field day with me then. I always had at least nine tasks in progress at any one time, all in the stratosphere, like a stack of aircraft waiting to land. Too many aircraft in the stack for too long and they run out of fuel.

Interesting thought.

All my aircraft had to land by nightfall, otherwise I'd failed. No wonder I was lagging and flagging.

Definition: The sign of a truly ailing workaholic is doing the housework in your underwear or leaving for the office before the streets are aired!

But rushing, frenzied workaholics don't stay healthy for long; they just have clinically clean houses or huge dry cleaning bills from being sprayed every day at six a.m. by those large machines which de-gunge the gutters and spew dirty water all over the sidewalk/pavement/road/street!

On the other side of the coin, you don't have to be a workaholic to be worn to a frazzle; but workaholics are the worst types for taking advice. They know it all. Their 'addiction' leads to exhaustion long before they realize there is a problem; I was a fully paid-up member.

Workaholism is the same as any other dependent habit — drink, drugs, cigarettes, chocolate, Armani coat hangers . . . Admitting the predicament is half-way to finding the cure.

According to Diane Fassel, in her book *Working Ourselves to Death*, workaholism is one of the most pervasive diseases of our society but also a progressive and potentially fatal disease. But because working hard, performing and achieving and coping without complaint are considered respectable activities, because workaholics are seen to be the ones 'getting ahead', the addiction is not taken seriously. In fact, the opposite is true. Slow down, adjust your performance level to suit your *health* and you could be accused, in some quarters, of not pulling your weight. And it's not just the province of big business. It's usual to associate workaholism with business suits and staying late at the office but, if you are the kind of person who simply cannot slow down and rest, you can be just as much a workaholic in any situation you care to name, in any walk of life, in any job and even during so-called leisure time.

Raising a family and keeping the home functioning is more than a full-time occupation but is one of the main areas of neglect. Neglect of ourselves in favour of our family duties. Why is it that looking after number one takes so little precedence?

Hang on a minute, here . . .

It's all very well telling people they should do less, not worry so much, leave everything in a shambles for the sake of their health. But what if not doing things makes them more stressed and more fretful? I understand that feeling too.

I once tried Shirley Conran's *Superwoman* strategy, gave up ironing the linen for a while, unco-ordinated the wardrobe and left the cupboards looking as if three cats and a dog had been fighting in them with the doors shut. I might have made a fortune as a fashion designer if I'd thought at the time that anyone would be remotely interested in the creased look as the latest catwalk couture. But crumpled grunge is not my scene – and it worried me even more than not ironing the bed (I'll tell you the bed-ironing story another time) – so I went back to ironing and cupboard tidying.

I did, however, make plenty of changes in other areas, made more time for eating healthily, resting regularly, exercising enjoyably and allowing an aircraft or two to land the next day instead – or even the day after that. Now old Tiredness only sneaks in if I overdo things and don't look after myself.

All Day Energy shares those discoveries with you. And they do make a difference, believe me, for all ages and both sexes, even the most stubborn amongst you who stick resolutely to 'I'm fine' when anyone asks how you are feeling. Fibber!

Complaints of fatigue and related symptoms are supposed to be one of the most common conditions that patients take to their doctors. And it seems to be true. In fact, I carried out a small study of my own into this sad state of affairs and found that, of new patients attending my clinic over a five-year period, around 92 per cent used words and phrases such as 'worn out', 'tired all the time', 'no energy', 'lethargic', 'exhausted', 'stressed', 'run out of steam'. Interestingly, improved energy levels were among the first comments reported at the follow-up consultation only a few weeks later.

My husband, Ralph, was another one who used to be plagued by tiredness and stress. Lack of energy became complete exhaustion but he didn't see the warning signs. Eventually, the cables snapped and he just couldn't take any more. His health deteriorated to the point where persistent indigestion became stomach cancer. Now that he has recovered and taken stock of his life, he finds that he worries far less about the trivia that would, once upon a time, have distressed him to distraction and irritated him into insomnia. Life-threatening illness can be sobering and enlightening.

He now enjoys life to the full and has tremendous energy but says that time passes so quickly, he seems to be constantly putting on or taking off his pyjamas! (So now you think he's a smouldering sexual athlete, huh? Well, since you mention it, he *is* more than a bit gorgeous – a work colleague of mine who saw a photograph of him recently thinks he looks 'tasty' – and he *has* got great legs, but don't get your hopes up. He's also loyal, faithful – and mine!)

Seriously, though . . .

He was a stressed, exhausted, overweight, edge of the seat all day, fall asleep in front of the TV at night, too tired to enjoy life, you guessed it – zombie. A better example of business executive stress leading to sickness you would have been unlikely to find. Proving that illness, tiredness and bouts of insecurity and hopelessness can attack at random – in any order – and affect the most confident of people. We happen to believe that one of the many reasons he got sick was because of what stress, overwork, poor diet and bottled-up emotions had done to him over a long period of years.

Added to all this, he felt directionless and inadequate.

Inadequate!

Unbelievable!

He was the one who taught *me* adequacy and self-reliance, who gave *me* the confidence to go out and give seminars to audiences of a thousand people at a time, to change from being a shivering brown mouse (yes, honestly, brown – see page 62!) into a comfortable introvert with extrovert bias.

But feeling below par plays havoc with one's perspective and will sometimes drag a person so far down that it can be difficult to turn around and climb back out of the pit. He made it – and so did I. You can too!

We realized – almost too late – that there is more to life than rush, rush, rush . . . crash. We realized, too, that there are no magic bullets but there are simple, sensible and enjoyable ways of finding out what ails you, taking action, boosting your energy, feeling great. If you sort out that nagging weight problem at the same time, that's a bonus.

All Day Energy is for *anyone* with an energy problem. It *isn't* a 'Don't do this, can't do that' instruction manual, full of negative comments and impossible-to-stick-to rules and regulations. It's a book full of tried and tested tips that you'll find simple, practical and cheerful. If you are overdue for a good chortle, then have one at my expense. I've discovered that laughing at oneself is excellent therapy. In addition to the wry smiles, you'll learn some of the more serious aspects of being tired all the time: how exhaust fumes can exhaust you; why too long in front of the VDU can make you lethargic; if you're a frequent flyer, why jetlag isn't inevitable and can be prevented; how mood and attitude can affect your health and your energy – and much, much more. You'll find out why some foods feed energy into the system and others sap it out. The section on Eating for Energy (page 257) will give you more information.

By the time you have learned to power up with *All Day Energy*, you'll enjoy feeling healthier, less likely to be laid low, energized and ready for anything.

When I asked one of my patients what she wanted most from her treatment, she told me 'I want to put the zip, zoom, bang, boom back into my life.' I guess that's where the inspiration for this book has come from.

Wishing you love and the best of health.

Kathryn Marsden
Wiltshire, England
January 1995

Introduction by Dr Tony Pickup

Few of us would deny the fact that illness at all levels — from simple headaches to more serious disorders — can be caused or exacerbated by the stress we experience in our modern world. We spend so much time 'doing' and then worrying about what we haven't done that there is never any time left for the real Self. Result? **Stress, lethargy, lack of energy** and a greater susceptibility to **malaise**. The most vicious of vicious circles.

With the best of intentions, most people have made at least some attempt to reduce their stress levels, take more exercise, lose some weight — but somehow their efforts were thwarted. It was all too difficult, there wasn't enough time, it didn't work. That kind of frustration has several outcomes — guilt, failure, anger, then more stress, followed by exhaustion and a kind of acceptance that there is nothing you can do to improve your situation.

Not true!

ALL DAY ENERGY is a comprehensive, no-nonsense book in which the reasons for feeling the way you do are explained in terms that everyone can relate to; some of them apply to all of us! Kathryn Marsden provides practical, non-judgemental solutions which enable the reader to make really positive changes, however limited their time or resources. Implement the advice where it applies to you and simply observe the effect. You should be very pleasantly surprised.

If you are under stress (who isn't?), Kathryn's first chapter will help you not only to assess the sources of that stress but also how to deal with them effectively. The problems of sleep are discussed in detail with tried and tested techniques to help the most vexed insomniac. There is an excellent chapter on the power of colour in our everyday lives – its message will CHANGE YOUR MOOD and LIFT YOUR ENERGY. For those fortunate – or unfortunate – enough to be flying (a stressful and exhausting activity in itself), there is a superb collection of strategies for protecting ourselves against the dreaded jet lag. If you suspect your chronic fatigue may be due to ME, the section on this thorny subject will give you guidance and encouragement.

Exercise and how to do it *properly* is given the prominence it deserves in *ALL DAY ENERGY* with sensible precautions against overdoing it! In this chapter you'll also find enjoyable stretching and relaxation techniques.

How to EAT HEALTHILY and to MAINTAIN A SENSIBLE WEIGHT are subjects addressed admirably in *ALL DAY ENERGY*. Medical systems the world over recognise the importance of good nutrition, many of them believing that a troubled digestive system is the root cause of most health problems. Our bodies have altered little in several thousand years – since the hunter-gatherer diet of fresh fruits, vegetables and occasional feasts of fresh game. And yet, modern nutritional advice and modern eating habits are only decades old. In evolutionary terms, the idea of 'meat and potatoes' is almost as recent as 'junk food'! Kathryn clouts a number of dietary misconceptions on the head and, in the process, takes the stress right out of 'healthy eating'. The chapters on EATING FOR ENERGY and her easy method of FOOD COMBINING should be read by everyone.

As you consume this book, you should find your stress dropping away, your eating becoming more enjoyable and your available energy increasing chapter by chapter.

Dr A.J. Pickup B.Sc (Hons), MRCS, LRCP, MFPM.

1

Why Do I Feel So Tired?

'Thinking is to me the greatest fatigue in the world.'
Sir John Vanbrugh (1664–1726)
The Relapse

Fatigue has many causes. Some kinds you can deal with, others you can't. The pleasurable exhaustion that comes after a long walk in the country (providing you didn't lose your way, drop your map in the mud and get all stressed out about which turning to take), an enjoyable (as opposed to excessive) workout session or a few hours flogging it round the flower beds; the odd late night, the lethargy associated with a bad cold or dose of influenza – such things will usually respond to a hot bath, a good night's sleep or a few days' rest and relaxation.

What about the other kind, though; the prolonged tiredness, the kind which never seems to go away? Sometimes, it's easy peasy to suss out the reasons behind fatigue; you don't need to be Sherlock Holmes or Dr Watson to see that burning the candle at both ends for too long (whether at work or play) is likely to put a strain on the system. Not so simple to figure are the cases where someone sleeps a regulation eight hours, who works but doesn't overwork and only burns candles during power failures. For them, their insidious accumulating exhaustion is a real puzzle.

And it isn't simply a matter of whether or not you are physically active. Many of us will, I'm sure, relate to the sentiments of the English dramatist and architect, Sir John Vanbrugh who found *thinking* fatiguing. Anyone who is involved with daily planning, organizing, creating and inventing (and that includes almost everybody) can get tired, even if their work is sedentary. Using the brain can be just as wearying as physical activity; indeed, when taken to extremes, an overactive mind can lead to severe stress and physical exhaustion.

For those who have spent years studying the effects of modern lifestyle on our health and energy levels, the conundrum is becoming clearer. Clinical observations, personal experience and evidence collected from patients have made me, for one, realize that chronic exhaustion can be brought on or aggravated by *many* different things; some all too obvious, others which may not, immediately, connect.

Such as?

How about, such as:

*** You're a touch overweight? (actually, four kilos and counting). That's a fairly obvious one. Dragging extra pounds around requires extra energy.

*** But you've been on every diet ever invented and (let me guess) none of them has worked long-term – and you're exhausted too? Did you know that dieting can drag your energy down? Don't give up on me here. I've some fairly strong things to say about crummy, useless, con-trick diets. Find out some of the best

---

ways to solve weight problems, safely and effectively – on page 257.

*** You're experiencing sleep deprivation better known as persistent lack of shut eye? You know you need more sleep but the best laid plans (no pun intended) for an early night never quite work out, do they? Learn how to turn on your sleep switch from page 89.

*** You work ridiculously, stupidly, excessively long hours?

*** You're stressed out of your mind?

*** The family has to come first?

*** You're bored with absolutely everything?

*** You worry too much about stuff?

*** Your mind is so overactive, your brain is on overtime? Pages 240–255 are where to go for the cures.

*** You eat terrible food (mostly takeaways and things out of packets and tins); I'm just wondering something here. Do they call them TV dinners because they taste like TV sets?

*** You eat everything too quickly?

*** You eat on the move? Fat chance *your* food has of being digested properly or at all, I'd say.

*** Your house / bedsit / apartment / studio / flat comes with cooking equipment but you haven't had time to fathom out how it works?

*** You have a lot of indigestion? *Indigestion can make you tired?* You'd better believe it! I'll tell you more from page 267.

*** You bought this book in an airport, so you probably spend a lot of your times in aeroplanes? Fix jetlag for good by following the tips on page 115.

*** Exercise. What's that? You don't do any, huh? Why not? You don't like it? See me for some special treatment – on page 219.

*** You are forced to breathe Foul and Filthy air – as in, you can't see across the street for the fumes or your air-con is on the blink and never serviced?

*** You spend great chunks of your day in front of a VDU?

*** You hardly see daylight or fresh air apart from the mad dash from your house to car to supermarket to office and back.

*** Your workplace has no windows, just loads of fluorescent lighting – and carpeting which gives you electric shocks? Improve your environment by reading pages 125 to 150.

*** Maybe you have an underactive (or overactive) thyroid gland. Whether this is just a suspicion or a firm diagnosis, page 157 should be of interest.

*** Perhaps your blood pressure is low. You thought low was healthy. Yes, mostly it is but if you are already under par, a low b.p. ain't so helpful. High blood pressure may be linked to fatigue too. If the info on page 154 sounds like you, take yourself off for a check-up.

*** You look unusually drawn. Could be anaemia. No, don't reach for the iron tablets just yet. Check with the doctor first. Tips on how to put the glow and colour back in your cheeks are scattered throughout *All Day Energy*.

*** Talking about colour, did you know that wearing the wrong colours can affect how you feel – and look? All will be revealed from page 57.

*** Your blood glucose levels seem to fluctuate more rapidly than the weather or the stock market? Could be hypoglycaemia, a common cause of energy loss – and you may not even realize you have it. Help for hypos begins on page 162.

*** A viral infection which should be long gone has clung to you like superglue to a blanket. Could be ME. No, not *me*. I mean M.E., Myalgic Encephalomyelitis, also known as Chronic Fatigue or Post-Viral Fatigue Syndrome. A real illness, not 'yuppy flu'. The person who thought up that stupid remark has obviously never had Chronic Fatigue Syndrome. Find the facts from page 183.

*** Candidiasis seems to be another important cause of fatigue. Encouragingly, symptoms can be much relieved by good dietary management and the right kind of anti-fungal supplements. More information is on page 201.

*** Bowel disorders including constipation, irritable bowel syndrome and colonic dysbiosis (disturbance of the balance of friendly flora in the gut) are commonly associated with lethargy and listlessness. If you are a sufferer, you should find *All Day Energy* has lots of helpful advice.

*** Tiredness may be caused or exacerbated by deficiency of one or more vitamins or minerals. Information on supplementation appears on page 307.

*** You keep yourself going with coffee, tea and chocolate fixes?

*** You eat lots of bread? Bread? What on earth has bread to do with fatigue? Trust me. Certain kinds of bread really do sap energy. So do some other foods, especially if your digestion isn't functioning top notch. That doesn't mean, though, that you have to give up bread. Find out more on page 280.

*** Some experts are convinced that allergies are a direct cause of fatigue. The dietary information on page 257 and the Energy and Environment chapter on page 125 should be helpful to anyone who suspects they may have food or environmental allergies.

And before we go any further, please note that where I use the word 'diet', this does not mean calorie-counted, deprived or depraved, sparing or slimming slop-in-a-glass abstinence. 'Diet' means nourishing, healthy, comestible, substantial sustenance which fills you, nurtures you, makes you feel good and gives you . . . ? YES! ENERGY!

So . . . the above list of possible tiredness-triggers isn't exhaustive (sorry, no pun intended here, either) but it does give you some idea how and why exhaustion is so common. It should also give you some encouragement to know that there is a healthy route to swapping exhaustion for energy.

If you are in the middle of any kind of upheaval just now, such as moving house, ironing the bed (I really will tell you that story some time), being busy on the job front, away from home, do-it-yourselfing, cleaning up after the do-it-themselfers, recouping after a spell in hospital or a bout of not-so-good health, you can still make a start on your ENERGY EVENT. Throughout the book, you'll find quick-to-read, quick-to-use LETHARGY LIFTERS that will begin to make a difference *right now.*

Right now, read on . . .

2

Power Up Against Stress

'In a disordered mind, as in a disordered body, soundness of health is impossible.'

Marcus Tullius Cicero
Roman orator, lawyer and statesman 106–43BC

Bones can crack under one sharp blow. Minds and bodies take longer. Attack a body and mind repeatedly with 'sharp blows' and, eventually, both will break under the strain. We've all seen it in others – many of us have come close to it ourselves.

Once upon a time, the words 'stress' and 'strain' applied only in the mechanical sense; engineering terminology and bridge-building boffins worrying about metal fatigue. Dr Hans Hugo Selye, the Austrian biochemist and founder of the Canadian Institute of Stress, is credited with being the first person to use the word 'stress' to describe mental and physical overload. Thanks to the work of Dr Selye (which began in the 1930s), the way stress affects our body is now fairly well understood.

I first read about his work in 1984 but even then, it seems, the stress/sickness link was not taken too seriously. During one of my many information-seeking nuisance raids, I raised this very point with a group of doctors (a profession well known for its high rates of breakdown, alcoholism, divorce and suicide, which works longer hours and suffers more stress and trauma than almost anyone else on this planet). I suggested that if people under stress were more likely to fall ill, wouldn't boosting the immune system reduce the risk? I didn't understand why I was thinking along these lines; something just told me it was commonsense.

Bold and fearless (some would say foolhardy), that was me – and with good reason. At about that time, what was left of my husband had just been discharged from hospital and I was pestering anyone and everyone about any possible links between diet, stress, immunity and the diagnosis of cancer in order to try to help him. He had *no right* to be stressed, of course. Stomach whipped out, then spleen, six weeks to live. No worries.

My theories were dismissed as 'unlikely'. Then guess what they told me?

'There's no scientific evidence . . .'

Nowadays, of course, stress and illness are synonymous. A stressed person is an exhausted person who is often also a sick person; falling ill creates more stress and so the cycle begins again. It has long been suggested that traumatic life events – such as bereavement, moving house or divorce – have direct or indirect connections with stress and the onset of health problems. Stress at work has now taken its (inevitable?) place on the list although I think most of us would say that we knew that already!

STRESS STUDIES

A company survey carried out in 1993 by the National Association for Mental Health found that problems at work could cause stress equal to, or possibly more than, that outside the workplace. Financial concerns, recession fear of redundancy and work pressure were named as the main causes of stress. Some firms believed that stress-related illness could be responsible for as much as 50 per cent of absenteeism. Stress-related headaches and migraine were singled out for special mention.

One study, carried out at the Churchill Hospital in Oxford, England, and reported in the *British Medical Journal*, appeared to debunk the idea that distressing events could be linked to ill health, at least in one specific area. The report says that women who suffer from severe stress were no more likely to have relapses of cancer than those women who were not under severe stress.

On the other hand . . .

Dr Guy Newell, author of *Stress and Cancer – The Interactions of Mind and Body*, concludes that the stress/cancer association has accumulated enough evidence to warrant more scientific enquiry.

Research also confirms a simple something that most of us have surely suspected for years – that serious stress can almost double the risk of going down with a cold. Additionally, being stressed can also prolong recovery time. The workaholic martyr who 'simply can't' take time off to recuperate is often the one who suffers from consecutive infections. 'Catching' one virus after another is nothing to be proud of if you're the nitwit passing it – ping-pong fashion – to everyone else within coughing and sneezing distance.

NEGATIVE STRESS

Stress, exhaustion, lack of confidence, low self-esteem and the wasted effort that people often expend in trying to secure the approval and goodwill of others can all be triggers for more stress.

There is no doubt about it, the 'S' word is surrounded by negative connotations. We associate it with illness, panic, upset, unhappiness, worry, nervous tension, having too much to do and feeling out of control. The result can be the same whether your angst is fuelled by a build-up of everyday hassles or a major event. You might have been word perfect in the mirror but come the examination, driving test or important meeting and your knees turn to jelly, your mouth dries, your thoughts race and you stumble over your sentences. In these kinds of situations, the panic of the experience is usually *inside you* and really doesn't show on the surface – even though you think you look like a shivering, blabbering, clammy incompetent. But that doesn't stop you from feeling terrible at the time and shattered after the event. When the initial panic is ended and calm washes over, you can still feel drained and exhausted.

For some people, the symptoms of stress can actuate some very unpleasant physical reactions. For example:

> Anxiety/panic attacks –
> which can, in turn,
> initiate attacks of asthma
> Churning stomach
> Cold hands or feet
> Difficulty breathing

Dizziness or fainting
Dry mouth
Fast heart beat
Feeling either chilled to the marrow or burning up
Headaches or migraine
Indigestion
Irritable bowel
Nausea
Profuse sweating
Raised blood pressure
Rapid pulse
Shaking
Skin flare-ups

It's highly unlikely that all these sensations and symptoms will manifest during every stressful episode or in every sufferer but experiencing only one or two can still be extremely unpleasant. Whether they are short-term or prolonged will depend upon the perceived severity of the stress as well as the individual response.

Skin conditions such as psoriasis and acne have long been associated with stress. Even warts (which are believed to have a viral connection) may be linked to anxiety in children and brought on by problems at school or disharmony at home. Viral infections have an opportunist streak and are more likely to attack those with a lowered immunity. Stress and anxiety are known to have a detrimental effect upon the immune system.

Studies at the University of Pittsburgh School of Medicine found that, although stress-related amenorrhea (absence of periods) is also associated with the underweight or over-exercised, as many as 50 per cent of cases could have a stress connection. Women taking part in the study could also link negative feelings to commonplace aggravation such as deadlines or arguments more often than they could to acute episodes of stress; proving that stress can be troublesome whether it comes in irritating trickles or great dollops. And if simple 'lack of periods' doesn't impress you as serious, bear in mind that abnormal menstruation is one of the leading causes of infertility.

SEX UNDER STRESS

For men, pressure at work, lack of self-esteem and fear of failure are common triggers for stress-related sexual problems. Premature ejaculation and 'erectile dysfunction' (also whispered as impotence) are said to be stress-linked in 60–70 per cent of cases. Stress can also reduce sperm count – and so affect fertility. 'A man ain't a man if he can't get it up', is the kind of emotional pressure that increases sense of failure and lack of confidence as well as reducing the chances of someone asking for help.

WOMEN MOST LIKELY TO . . .

According to surveys carried out by the National Center for Health Statistics, women are more likely to feel that stress has affected their health and are twice as likely to seek help for their problems. We know that this doesn't mean men don't get stressed, of course, but hunky homosap does seem to be more reluctant to show his

feelings or discuss his symptoms; he sees them as weaknesses. Whingeing, whether of the pom or any other
variety, is a pain in anybody's language but there has to
be a middle ground between complaining all the time
about everything that ails you and saying you're fine when
you clearly are not.

A TROUBLE SHARED REALLY IS A TROUBLE HALVED

So much stress can be caused by misunderstandings, too.
If people don't say how they feel or share what is troubling
them, they can actually create more stressful situations for
other people who want to help but are being frozen out.

STRESS IS . . .

Another angle on stress came to light while I was
researching this book and interviewing people about their
perception of stress. Several women expressed the view
that they became stressed when they felt obliged to sort
out the shambles created by other people who didn't
appear to suffer from stress at all.

> *'Stress,' said one, 'is so often the consequence of suppressing
> the burning desire to choke the living daylights out of some
> disorganized and irritating individual who desperately
> needs a kick up the trousers.'*

Husbands and children were mentioned. Strange that!

ARE YOU BOTHERED BY STRESS?

The following comments are some of the most common ones uttered by patients who are affected by stress and lack of energy. Reading through the list can help a stressed person to identify some of the stressors in their professional and personal life. Acknowledging that there is a problem in a particular area can provide the impetus either to change the situation or alter the attitude towards it. Learning to reduce the stress can, in itself, help to restore the lost energy.

You'll see that each phrase is accompanied by A, B or C.
'A' = this is definitely you
'B' = this sounds like you every now and then
'C' = No problem
Read the list quickly, don't linger. Put a circle around the letters which apply to you. Above all, be honest; otherwise there is little point in doing the quiz. I'll leave you to work out the scores for yourself!

I have too many responsibilities	A	B	C
I set high standards for myself	A	B	C
I expect high standards of others	A	B	C

I'm always involved in confrontation	A	B	C
I worry about being late for appointments	A	B	C
I'm always late for appointments	A	B	C
I hate driving	A	B	C
Other drivers annoy me	A	B	C
I hate being in a queue	A	B	C
I smoke to calm my nerves	A	B	C
I drink to calm my nerves	A	B	C
I get angry easily	A	B	C
I hate the way I look	A	B	C
I hardly ever laugh	A	B	C
I don't smile much	A	B	C
I'm not very good at my job	A	B	C
I make a lot of mistakes	A	B	C

My job is monotonous/boring/ unchallenging	A	B	C
I am intimidated by authority	A	B	C
I must work to deadlines	A	B	C
I'm hassled all the time	A	B	C
I hate my boss	A	B	C
I have difficulty saying 'No' to people	A	B	C
I feel taken for granted	A	B	C
Family problems are always left to me	A	B	C
Everyone uses me	A	B	C
There's never enough time	A	B	C
I'm sure people don't like me	A	B	C
Nobody loves me	A	B	C
Nobody listens to my opinions	A	B	C
I'm tired most of the time	A	B	C

My work takes me away from home
too much   A   B   C

I'm nervous about meeting new
people   A   B   C

I'm always trying to please everyone   A   B   C

I find it difficult to concentrate   A   B   C

I'm always in a hurry   A   B   C

I never have any time to myself   A   B   C

I get impatient easily   A   B   C

I run out of steam quickly   A   B   C

I feel lethargic most of the time   A   B   C

I am easily frightened or panicked   A   B   C

I feel tearful quite a lot of the time   A   B   C

I sleep badly   A   B   C

I feel like a worn out rag first thing
in the morning   A   B   C

I find it difficult to concentrate   A   B   C

My life moves along at a frantic pace	A B C
I feel restless when sitting still	A B C
I worry a lot	A B C
I bite my nails and nibble at the skin	A B C
Feeling stressed makes me breathless	A B C
Something always needs doing	A B C
Stress gives me indigestion	A B C
My neck aches	A B C
I'm bored	A B C
I overeat	A B C
I have no appetite	A B C
I worry about what people think of me	A B C
I worry excessively about my health	A B C
I worry excessively about my finances	A B C
Now I'm worried because my answers are mostly 'A's	A B C

How did you get on with that lot? OK? Good. Not so great? A bit revealing was it? Don't worry about it. You are definitely not alone here. With a bit of help and a good laugh, you'd be amazed at how much better you are going to feel.

DEFINING STRESS

The dictionary definition confirms *stress* as 'Constraining or compelling effort'. Interestingly, the same entry explains that mechanical stress can lead to metal fatigue.

So why should people be any different?

Now you know why your mechanical bits are feeling a mite rusty here and there. They are probably overtired, overused and in need of a service.

The difference between machines and people is that people also have hearts, souls and spirits – which can also be battered and broken (in other words, stressed) by excessive wear and tear. When the body and mind can no longer function properly because they haven't been allowed to repair and rejuvenate, the result is collapse. Your system is shouting for help but because you either don't hear or aren't listening, it shuts down and makes you take a break whether you like it or not. That's what happened to me, why I collapsed all those years ago with exhaustion. I didn't understand what was happening at the time but I understand it now.

Whether stress is positive or negative depends upon how you look at it. One person's ambitious objective can be another person's panic attack. You use stress either as a plus or a minus. But you don't need me to tell you that. Dr Selye defined negative stress as *dis*-stress and positive stress as *eu*-stress. However you, personally, are affected by stress, one thing is for sure . . .

. . . STRESS USES ENERGY

Almost any change in routine or environment could be classed as 'stressful'. Some of life's greatest pleasures are stressful – but in a positive way. For example, surprise happenings, falling in love, achieving that hard-won promotion. Excitement, stimulation, anticipation, looking forward to something instead of dreading it – these emotions can be constructive and productive. It's normal to feel elated and then exhausted because of an exciting event – you are, after all, still using up energy; the difference is that such experiences make you feel better about yourself and your life. If your cells are happy and functioning as they should, your energy is soon restored.

A sudden shock, a threat to your safety or being unwell can trigger very similar physiological processes within the body to the positive experiences we mentioned a moment ago. They also use up masses of energy. From both extremes, the body has the power to recover fully.

The real danger occurs when the stress reaction is prolonged, when you remain on red alert and can't recuperate even after the threat has passed or, still more alarmingly, *when the person suffering from chronic stress isn't aware of the mounting danger*. When you are under persistent and unrelenting stress, it's easy to switch off the alarm and to keep going for quite a considerable time before meltdown becomes inevitable.

I call it the *Coiled Spring Syndrome*.

Impossible to unwind.

In fact, it is a useful analogy to see the coiled spring for what it really is – a loop of metal which, under persistent strain, becomes fatigued and snaps. Just like people do when they have used up all their energy reserves, have no resistance left to protect themselves and so, *just can't take it any more*. Even someone who swears that they thrive on positive stress can fall prey to breakdown if they never slow down. Perhaps we should all have a motto which reminds us to 'Take a break before we break'.

NO-ONE IS COMPLETELY IMMUNE

Everyone is touched by stress – good and bad. It's an unavoidable factor in our daily lives. Making banal comments about preventing or evading stress is pretty useless. Not many of us are in a position to simply dump our responsibilities; nor would most of us want to if we are completely honest. A desert island existence may seem attractive but so are the home comforts we take so much for granted. Anyhow, removing all stimulation and ambition could be as unhealthy as being overstressed. Running away is something most of us consider from time to time – usually when things are going badly, when we are tired, under pressure, frustrated, not feeling too well. When life proceeds smoothly and everything is 'cool running', our perspective changes.

OPTI-PESSI-MISM

It isn't necessarily true that optimists have less stress than pessimists but perhaps they deal with it more effectively and recover from it more easily. Getting the balance right between optimism and pessimism is what counts. We all know Mr or Mrs Professional Pessimist whose conversation revolves constantly around bad news. They regale you with depressing tales of someone's illness, yesterday's accident on the highway, nuclear disaster and the end of the world as we know it. You never ask them how they are unless you really want to hear lengthy chapter and verse about their latest bout of food poisoning, their bowel movements and their full, unabridged history of every hospital visit they've made since the Civil War. Not surprising, is it, that these gloom and doom merchants can make you stressed and anxious.

Take some advice.

Cross the street if you see them coming!

The Overly Optimistics, who live next door, may seem a better option but can be dreamers who believe that everything always gets better, rather than worse. Their major problem is that they can be easily put upon by others, seeing good in everybody, always happy to help and never complaining. They can also be knocked very badly by trauma if it affects them directly and unexpectedly.

Somewhere in between is the balance which takes a positive attitude towards everyday happenings but is also able to deal with the darker side of human behaviour and existence when it occurs. I do believe it is true that many of those who suffer from stress do so because they see

24

themselves as needing to remedy the problems caused by people who don't suffer from stress. Think about it.

A psychologist at the University of California Los Angeles has recently come up with the suggestion that wellbeing, at least in part, could be in our genes and that some people may be born with a predisposition towards happiness and contentment. (I can think of one or two who were definitely born with miserable genes.) But joy and gladness also depend upon which cards you are dealt and what you choose to do with your life. By adopting activities that are purposeful and by taking a positive attitude, it is possible to improve mood and see things in a constructive light.

FIGHT THE FOE OR RUN LIKE HELL?

Understanding the stress reaction can help a lot towards damage limitation. Dr Selye and his researchers concluded that when people experienced stress, their reactions followed a common pattern. You've heard of the Fight or Flight Syndrome – well, this is it:

When the body first perceives the *stressor*, chemical and electrical messengers are released and hormones are triggered. Your blood pressure, pulse rate and heartbeat all increase (palpitations seem familiar, do they?), blood thickens, lungs take in more air, digestion shuts down, muscles tense up (neck ache? headache?), your whole system is on red alert. All fine and dandy if you are needing to deal with immediate danger or challenge – such as a sabre-toothed tiger suddenly turns up uninvited in your back yard – but not so great if you're simply late for an appointment and someone holds you up in a lane of traffic.

Luckily, your hair stands on end when you are stressed, angry or frightened – an evolutionary throwback which is supposed to terrify your enemy. Very useful if you're having a bad day with the boss/partner/children. 'We'd better behave ourselves today – just look at Mother's hair!'

Your body will remain in this state of alert for as long as the perceived 'threat' persists. Trouble is, the sufferer can't always determine when the need to be under stress has passed. A perilous pattern then emerges. Whilst short-term stress in a healthy body should not present any problems, prolonged pressure can have a significantly detrimental effect upon the immune system, leaving you at greater risk of attack – this time by illness. And it doesn't usually happen overnight. More likely, bouts of ill health can creep up on you unawares and you may not even think to connect them with the stress you've been suffering for years.

Let the stress persist unabated and you become exhausted. Your adrenal system is still producing hormones which are, this time, trying to damp down the stress reaction. Unfortunately, one in particular – cortisol – further suppresses the immune system. This is the kind of chronic, long-term stress which is normally associated with serious illness.

But every increase in stress is related to an increase in risk, say researchers. Studies at Ohio State University showed that both short-term stress (such as exams, for example) and long-term stress (serious illness, caring for a loved one with chronic disease) caused a lowering of the body's immune defences.

If you know someone who is 'hyper' and finds difficulty winding down after a stressful experience, it's possible that their body is locked into alert mode. Normal body mechanisms are unlikely to be restored when a stressed system stays on permanent standby.

STRESS IS ON THE INCREASE

Exhaustion and lethargy appear to be affecting almost everyone.

Our health and well-being, despite many technological breakthroughs in medicine and science, seem to be on the decline.

Learning to understand and deal with stressful situations is, surely, more important than ever.

THINK POSITIVELY

It is possible to strengthen the system against stress attack, to lessen the risk of damage, to protect yourself so that when you are under threat, the effects dissipate quickly and you recover safely.

Experts believe that vulnerability to stress develops from learned behaviours and attitudes. It isn't the event that is inherently stressful but your perception of it. That's good news because it means that, given the right frame of mind, stress can become a challenge rather than something which rules and ruins your life. Positive thought has a lot going for it.

Cherie de Haas, a practitioner and friend who lives and works in Melbourne, always reminds her patients that *pressure* is what it takes to turn carbon into diamonds. It's OK to *POWER UP* as long as you learn to *POWER OFF*. Leaving the power switched on all the time uses up energy. Eventually, the energy runs out and you are exhausted – and, most probably, more stressed as a result.

That's what *All Day Energy* is all about: side-stepping negative stress, powering up to the positive stuff and showing you how to power off before the pressure builds to danger level.

TIME OUT

One of the primary obstacles to good *stress* management is poor *time* management. Another is allowing ourselves to be intimidated, held to ransom, by other people's needs. Two of the strongest associations with negative stress are 'There isn't enough time' and 'I'll feel guilty if I don't do X, Y and Z for So-and-So.'

Wound yourself very neatly into another vicious circle, hmmmm? You don't have enough time to pace yourself properly and do things for *you* but you're always available when someone *else* shouts. The boss, the neighbour, the spouse, the offspring. They are all well practised in the art of emotional blackmail.

'Could you just . . . ?'

'It'll only be for an hour or two . . .'

or the creepy crawly version of

'I just *had* to ask you because you're so *capable*.' Yuck! You know they are being nauseatingly insincere but somehow, well . . . it's easier to adopt a robot-mode 'compliance' than to say 'No'.

No?

Perish the thought.

Did you see the robot in the film *Short Circuit*? Known as 'Number Five', his willingness to agree, 'compliance' – and the pressure he was put under by his uncaring 'bosses' – eventually caused both his metal body and his human-like mind to shatter under stress. His 'body' was restored with the help of some new spare parts but his mind was repaired using tender loving care.

PUSHOVER PRESSURE

The inability to say 'NO' is surely one of the greatest health hazards. Unfortunately, most of us are pushovers for a favour. The good egg who is always available, no matter what the event and no matter how inconvenient it may be for us to drop everything and BE THERE. Of course, our readiness to comply may also be because we are afraid of what people might think of us if we say 'No'. There goes that word again. Isn't it easier to say yes and feel resentful than to say no and feel guilty?

You're sure you can hear them whispering.

'You know *thing* across the street? Well, I only asked if she could collect the kids from school, give them their tea, take them to the park, then read them a story, put them to bed, do the laundry, take out the garbage and sweep the chimney and guess what? She said "NO"! Can you believe anyone being that *unreasonable*?'

There is, absolutely and unequivocally, no need (hear

me out there? *no need*) to feel guilt or shame at, every now and then, saying you aren't available. If you are already exhausted, your health may depend upon it. There's no need to be aggressive or abrupt because you choose to say 'No'. Try softening the refusal by, first of all, using the person's name. 'It's really nice of you to think of me and I wish I could help; unfortunately, I'm just not available on those dates.' You don't have to give details. Or try 'I'd love to do that for you but there's something else booked for that day that I just can't change. Perhaps next time?'

You'll earn more respect if you choose not to be a wimp – and the ones who pressured you will see what an amazingly talented and popular person you really are. No, I'm not kidding. Too many people spend their time putting themselves down and being someone else's doormat. If you say 'No' to them, it must be because you have better fish to fry. Then you'll hear a different kind of whisper: 'I just *couldn't* bother her, she's *so* much in *demand*.'

Rarity value does funny things to people!

LET UP AND LET GO

Still too much to do and no time to do it? Here are a whole heap of things that can help to lighten your load. See which ones fit best into your lifestyle and then introduce one positive change at a time. It's useful, too, to read through the complete list regularly. Stress has a nasty habit of seeping into the system and sapping your energy, almost unnoticed; it's easy to slip back into old habits.

*** *Aromatherapy massage* is a wonderful de-stressor as well as having an established track record for helping a wide range of health problems. Remember that gentle massage is best for relaxation. Deep massage is more useful if you are treating a muscle spasm. Some of the key essential oils used in aromatherapy are, I believe, also essential additions to anyone's First Aid cabinet. Lavender, for example, soothes minor scalds and burns but its aroma is also very calming and relaxing – so great for de-stressing and encouraging sound sleep. Clary Sage, Frankincense and Sandalwood are also good for slowing down a stress freak.

Make a regular appointment for a full body massage. Listen and learn from the therapist and ask him or her to recommend some oils for you to use at home. (Never apply neat oils directly to the skin.) And remember, aromatherapy massage can put the zest back into your lovelife! Pick up a book on essential oils and familiarize yourself with the basics. The Further Reading list on page 340 has some excellent self-help titles.

*** Another *relaxing* therapy is *reflexology*, the massage of specific points on the feet, ankles and, sometimes, on the hands and face. Far from being 'quack' medicine, reflexology and aromatherapy have been practised the world over for thousands of years. To find a good practitioner, one of the best ways is to listen to the recommendations of other people who are pleased with the treatment they have received. In addition, Products and Services — on page 352 — will tell you how to go about finding a therapist in your area.

*** *Look after your feet*. Keep toenails cut and cleaned. Massage the feet each day with an oil or body lotion. Avoid talcum powder; it creeps into crevices and traps moisture, increasing the risk of infections. Don't be tempted into wearing punishing shoes just because they are supposed to be the height of fashion. Any kind of pain or discomfort will increase stress levels and could affect physical health too. The Chinese believe that each area of the foot relates to an area of the body, connected by a system of invisible energy lines. If your shoes pinch your toes, headaches and neck pain could be the result. I met one lady who told me she had suffered from blocked sinuses only when she wore a particular pair of boots. After a while, she realized that the footwear was chafing the area around her toes which related to her sinuses. Uncomfortable shoes are also said to be the quickest way to crow's feet (around your eyes)! If your feet hurt, it shows first in your face!

The orthodox medical profession has a hard time believing in such treatments and few doctors seem keen to recommend them, although attitudes are changing. However, there is no doubt that this therapy has helped a great many people to overcome a range of health problems; stress and insomnia would appear to respond particularly favourably and with none of the unpleasant side effects which have been associated with some painkillers, sleeping drugs and tranquillizers.

*** *Take a deep, relaxing bath*. Use your chosen oils and avoid adding ordinary soap (which can destroy the benefits of the oils themselves and also disturb the natural pH of your skin). But don't soak for too long at too high a temperature. Hot baths can put a strain on the circulation and lead to dehydration and dizziness. Excessive heat can also age the skin! Enjoying a moderately warm bath for no longer than ten minutes is the best way to wind down after a hard day.

*** Invest in a cassette tape of natural sounds – birdsong, a waterfall, wind in the trees, etc. Researchers have found that *listening to the sounds of nature can help to reduce stress and fatigue, and increase energy and alertness.* Whenever possible, get out into the countryside and tune into the real thing. Interestingly, some companies have invested in equipment that generates natural sounds and natural aromas into the workplace and have found employees to be more alert and less fatigued as a result.

*** Check out the possibility that *geopathic stress* may be aggravating anxiety or illness. For more information, see page 104 in the chapter on

Sleep or turn to Products and Services on page
349.

*** *See a chiropractor or an osteopath* for a
check-up. Head and neck pain, shoulder stiffness,
back problems, poor sleep pattern and a range of
other conditions can be caused or exacerbated by
spinal misalignment. A twice-yearly visit is well
worth while and should be considered a health
investment. Details on page 353.

*** Invest, also, in a copy of *Are You Sitting
Comfortably* by Andrew Wilson for valuable information on how to improve *posture*, reduce pain,
avoid RSI (repetitive strain injury), choose the right
work station and chair – and more. Details in the
Further Reading section on page 343.

*** *Transcendental Meditation* (TM) is
known to be helpful in the management of stress
and relief of anxiety. Regular practice is most beneficial. Turn to page 89 (the Sleep chapter) and
pages 339 and 357 (Further Reading and Products
and Services) for more information on classes and
books on the subject.

*** Consider having a 'make-over'. Visiting the
health spa or beauty salon for a restyle, a facial,
massage and manicure can do wonders for your
self-esteem and confidence. 'Treating yourself' is
often seen as extravagance. It is, in fact, an essential part of learning to *appreciate your own
value*. Read the chapter on Colourful Energy –
page 57.

*** *Regular exercise* is an important step in stress recovery. This does not, however, mean that you have to run a marathon each day before breakfast, swim ten miles before nightfall or work yourself into a sweaty blob at your local gym. The right level of exercise is known to help increase energy; overdoing it has the reverse effect. See page 219 for more info.

*** *Music* is valuable as a de-stressor. Relaxation tapes are widely available. Alternatively, your own favourites of popular or classical pieces will do just as well. The important thing is that the music you choose must be enjoyable and relaxing for *you*. A friend of mine who confesses to 'hating housework', finds that she actually enjoys it when she cleans 'to joyful music'.

*** *Programme your leisure time in advance.* Don't look upon relaxation and recreation as luxuries; they are vital contributors to a healthy lifestyle. It's not enough to assume that you might have a few minutes' unwinding time at the end of the day if you're not too busy. Make sure you plan your free time as carefully as you would a business appointment.

*** Cope with stress and curb your energy expenditure by setting *realistic goals* for yourself. Be aware of your strengths and weaknesses and be the best that you can be within your own boundaries. Don't feel that you always have to win or that you failed if you didn't come out on top every time.

Don't use phrases such as 'I must' or 'I have to' but 'I will if I can'.

*** *Solitude* can be an important contributor to relaxation and de-stressing. If you are totally unused to 'quality solitude', it can be a strange feeling. Scary stuff – coming face to face with yourself. Sometimes, people can be afraid of isolation from others because they think they might be lonely – but solitude is as far away from loneliness as silk is from sacking. Being alone sometimes helps to clarify thought and transform a foggy outlook, to see things that you might otherwise have missed in the daily rush and bustle. But don't be alone too much. Strike a balance so that you can benefit from your quiet times without cutting yourself off from your friends.

*** If you are feeling low, *be with people who care* about your wellbeing. It's a truism that in times of plenty your 'friends' will find you but in times of adversity you find your genuine friends. When you are down, support often comes from the most unexpected sources. Even though you might want to crawl away and hide, research shows that people do cope better with stress when they have the empathy and company of others.

And it doesn't have to be human. Pets are often very intuitive to people's emotions and needs. Talking to your cat or dog doesn't mean you're crazy. When Ralph was in hospital, our cat Emily searched for him every day. As soon as he came home to convalesce, she installed herself in the bedroom and stayed with him constantly. Ralph found her company enormously therapeutic. Once he was up and around, she went back to her normal routine. Some years later, when she died and we cried, our other cats definitely seemed to understand. We huddled together and shared our grief – and were all helped by one another. Anyone who sees that as crazy behaviour may have a serious problem of their own!

*** *Don't be afraid to cry.* It's a fact of life that women tend to cry more easily; most men cling dutifully to the macho image which says that stiff upper lips are *de rigueur*. That doesn't mean men don't *feel* like crying or don't hide away and howl in private. Why do you think they go through the 'pull yourself together', 'you shouldn't let things get to you', 'what are you blubbing about now?' routine? Could it be because they are afraid that they might be affected by your emotions? In fact, telling people to 'pull themselves together' is neither helpful nor endearing and can even be harmful.

Shedding tears every now and then is not wimpish. On a purely physical level, the lubrication in the eyes supplies oxygen to the cornea of the eye and carries away carbon dioxide and waste debris. On an emotional level, releasing tears releases stress, discharging the 'toxic' burden that trauma and anxiety puts on the system. The actual fluid contains hormones which, if kept bottled up, could prolong your depression and perpetuate your unhappiness.

When you cry, you may feel washed out for a while afterwards but it is uncanny how much less distorted your thought processes suddenly become after a good sobbing session.

*** ***Don't be embarrassed about showing emotion*** either during or after a traumatic, distressing or frightening occurrence. Far from being a sign of weakness, expressing how you feel is the body's intelligent response to 'dis-stress'.

*** ***Don't suffer in silence.*** If you need help, ask. Seek out a supportive colleague, a good friend – or a professional. If you are plagued by sexual difficulties, remember that psychosexual counselling is available via most GPs' surgeries.

*** ***Walk out in the fresh air*** – every day if you can. Natural light is known to improve mood. Breathe, look around you, let your mind wander but, above all, forget about work.

*** Reduced light levels during the winter months are known to cause fatigue, irritability, depression, poor concentration, appetite disturbance, anxiety and stress in some people. If this sounds like you, take whatever steps you can to ***lighten and brighten your*** internal ***surroundings.*** Bring plants into your home, choose paint, wallpaper, curtains and other furnishings in light reflecting colours. Avoid blue; it can flatten your mood even further if you are already feeling that way. Check out the chapter on Colourful Energy for more information (page 57).

Ordinary fluorescent lighting (you'll recognize it at once – it's the level of light designed to make humans look like luminous 'aliens') is almost impossible to avoid; just try to spend as little time under its devastating glare as possible.

Whenever you can, work near to a window. Get yourself outside into the fresh air and daylight for half an hour every day – even when the weather is not so good and the sky is overcast – but especially when the winter sun breaks through.

*** A much more serious version of the 'winter blues' is a condition akin to hibernation called *SAD – Seasonal Affective Disorder* – where reduced levels of daylight during the winter months cause severe depression often accompanied by lethargy, a need for excessive sleep, lack of sex drive, irritability and weight problems.

Once spring has sprung, SAD depression lifts and symptoms disappear. As you'll find when you read the chapter on Sleep (page 89), lack of natural light can cause serious disruption to our body clocks and, in turn, to our long term health. SAD used to be treated with drug medication but in recent years, researchers have discovered that exposure to full spectrum lighting (which mimics daylight) can bring quite dramatic and beneficial improvements. If you have been diagnosed with SAD, you may find a full spectrum 'light box' installed in your home or office a real health investment. Full details of support groups and suppliers are on pages 354–355.

*** ***Deep breathing*** exercises not only de-stress, they help transport valuable oxygen around your exhausted body. Without oxygen, we die. People who don't breathe properly are not feeding their cells with sufficient oxygen (or shedding toxins efficiently) so you could say that they are dying slowly. In the chapter on Energy and Exercise (page 219), you'll find a number of beneficial breathing techniques.

*** ***Try yoga***, ***tai chi*** or other ***meditation.*** If you think this is the province of the weirdo brigade, you're wrong. Join a class and you'll find real people, probably with similar problems, and not a bed of nails in sight. Your local library, Adult Education centre or Community College will hold information on classes in your area.

*** ***Aim to get out of your bed 15 minutes earlier in the morning*** and, if possible, use this extra space for yourself and no-one else. Those few extra minutes of 'pottering time' can make the difference between a frantic day and an enjoyable one.

*** ***Wake up slowly.*** Choose a user-friendly system of starting the day. If you can't come round without a reminder, a radio alarm with a clock display and a gentle repeated facility is less jarring and kinder to your adrenalin production than a loud buzzer or bell which blasts your brain into the stratosphere every morning.

*** ***Take short breaks throughout the day*** to recharge your batteries. Even a minute or two away from the desk or outside the house or office can make a huge difference to your daily reserves of energy. Never attempt to work through the whole day without some kind of diversion.

*** *Take definite meal breaks*, preferably away from your working area. Eating at the desk or on the move can wreak havoc with your digestive system and reduce the amount of nourishment you are likely to absorb from your food. Breakfast meetings and business lunches may be an acceptable part of corporate life but that doesn't mean they are healthy.

*** *Avoid racing and rushing.* Few of us ever leave enough time when dashing from one venue to another. For every appointment you make, add ten or fifteen minutes so that, say, for an 11 o'clock meeting, you write down 10.50 a.m. That way, you're more likely to arrive on time. I know some people who set their wrist watches and clocks accordingly! Consequently, they are never rushed, never late and they stay calm.

*** It's worth repeating the old Chinese proverb which says that the palest ink is better than the most retentive memory. When you are under pressure, your brain cells don't always function at their best and you find yourself forgetting things more easily. So carry a notepad and *write things down* when they pop into your head. Or do what I do and carry a mini memo recorder in your pocket or purse. An idea, something for the shopping list, an appointment – I just tell my pocket memo. At the end of the day, I rewind and listen to my messages and enter them into my diary only if necessary. (I have to tell you a quick story here. Ralph asked me what I would like for my birthday and I said anything would do as long as it didn't have a plug on it – for a change. So he bought me my pocket memo – something which works on batteries!)

*** *Get to know which factors in your life cause you anxiety* (the questionnaire on pages 16–20 will help you to identify some of these). When things happen that you don't feel so good about, note them down. At the end of the month, check the list and see if there are any common denominators. For example, if you find that 'traffic jams on the way to work' appears more than once on your list, then this may be an area which is causing you particular concern. Until you wrote it down, you may not even have realized that it was a problem. Could you overcome this area of hassle by taking a different route, opting for flexitime, leaving home earlier (or later) in the morning or altering your hours in some other way?

*** Steal this idea from an American I met mid-Atlantic on the *QE2*. (I was working – he was on vacation!) Once in a while, he tells me, work on Saturday morning and *take half a day off during the week.* OK, I can hear you. 'This is going to help me reduce my stress?' It could do. It could be fun to feel self-righteous about working on the weekend when everyone else is off duty. It often means you get through more work than you would on a regular day. It can also feel great to take a day off midweek when everyone else is slogging it! A treat especially for you.

*** *Be a bit better organized.* Being prepared for emergencies means that if an emergency comes along, it won't be an emergency and you won't become all stressed up about it – if you see what I mean. For a start, why not lighten that trolley load of junk you call a briefcase/handbag and empty out the crinkle sprockets, sweet wrappers and widgets? (When did you last need to take a boy scout out of a horse's hoof, anyway?) Replace the widgets with really useful items. Invest in a make-up pouch and keep in it a new pair of tights or stockings (they take up no room at all if you remove all the cardboard and fold them in a mini polythene bag), a sticking plaster, a mini sewing kit (hotels give them away), a nail file, cards or coins for the telephone, a few stamps, a notepad, a pen or pencil, a booklet of *papier poudre* (paper tissue sheets impregnated with shine-removing face powder), a pouch-sized Evian spray, a lipstick and tissues in a travel pack. You may have other things you can add to the list but you get the general idea. None of them weighs heavy and they could save you from disaster.

*** Prevent the irritation which is so often caused by a faulty piece of equipment by *getting it fixed!*

*** *Think ahead to save yourself some hassle.* Always leave a pen and pad by the phone. Fill your petrol tank before you reach the 'panic, panic, warning light is flashing' stage. Keep the first aid box up-to-date and have some spare light bulbs in the house. In case there is a power failure, put candles, candle holders, a torch and matches where you can find them easily.

*** Whenever possible, try to complete the 'I'm not so keen on this' sort of jobs earlier in the day so that you can *look forward to the tasks you really do enjoy.* You'll find this especially helpful on 'down' days.

*** *Get plenty of sleep.* Seems an obvious thing to say but it's surprising how many of us try to exist on too little.

*** *Plan the week's menu* before you do the weekly shopping; it may appear to take up more time but actually saves time and trouble as the week progresses. There is no last minute panic about 'what to have for dinner' *and* you could spend less at the store.

*** In case you didn't get the message earlier on in this chapter, *remember that it's OK to say 'No' sometimes.*

*** *Stop and stare.* Do nothing every now and then. There is a maxim which says 'Accomplishing nothing can often result in mission accomplished.'

*** It's said that those who can't delegate are bad managers. Whether this is true or not, *lighten the* *load* by letting someone else help *you* out now and then.

*** *Laugh* – it really is good medicine. It activates deeper breathing, improves the circulation and can improve your blood pressure and heart rate too. Don't grow old with your mouth turned down at the corners. There are already too many unhappy people in the world. There are also a few who seem to make a career out of being miserable and knocking anything and everything positive that anyone else tries to do. If *they* laughed, their faces would probably crack! Try to see the funny side of situations and don't take everything so seriously.

Have you ever noticed how laughter can suddenly interrupt an attack of anger? A good giggle can be a very healthy release from tension, stress, embarrassment and lethargy. A sense of humour is also said to strengthen the immune system. According to a cable tv cartoon network in America, almost 20 per cent of its viewers are women over the age of eighteen. Fans say that cartoons are a way of escaping from life's pressures; it seems that Tom, Jerry, 'Shylveshter', Popeye and Bugs Bunny have the power to lift mood far more effectively than comedy shows which can be too 'issue-oriented' by politics, sex, religion, etc.

*** *Skip the headlines.* For at least one day a week, don't turn on the tv or radio news. Subscribe to a publication which publishes only upbeat, easy on the mind, news. Read comic strips or silly stories about underwater hang-gliding and two-piece jig-saw puzzles. Take a suggestion from one of my former patients who, during her recovery from ME, cancelled her *Literary Supplement* and changed to a glossy picture magazine.

*** Collect *wacky cartoons.* I have one of my favourites taped to my desk which reminds me 'Why cats are better than men.' My husband loves it:

1. They think they look wonderful in the morning. (Cat landing enthusiastically on the bed, knocking the wind out of your lungs.)

2. They take an interest in your work. (Cat sitting on top of computer with front paws draped over the screen.)

*** Have you ever noticed how some people can make you feel cheerful and others can bring on black depression. If possible – and especially when you are not well or are already overtired, try to *avoid people who dwell on misery.* I call them 'button-holers'. They pin you down, create mountains out of mole-hills, talk about themselves and never pause for breath. They might ask you how you are but then talk over your answer. Their negative energies can drain you and leave you feeling even more exhausted. Mix with relaxed, non-worriers instead.

*** *Check your breathing.* Are you taking deep breaths? Don't forget how helpful that can be in a stressful situation.

*** *Sort your needs from your necessities.*

Having enough to eat, being clothed, being warm (or cool) enough and having enough money to put a few pennies by and pay your bills – those are necessities. Anything else that comes along is a bonus not a stress!

*** ***Buy yourself a piggy bank.*** Feed it with your smallest of small change. Then empty it once a month or once a year and use the money to treat yourself; not the kids or your mother – you. Movie tickets, a video, a cream cake, a visit to your favourite gallery, a plant from your local nursery or garden centre, a bottle of bubbly, some new writing paper, a book – something personal for you.

*** If someone makes you angry, you can still avoid the argument without bottling up the stress. I once worked with a fella who had the perfect answer to this problem. He said 'Wait twenty-four hours and then think about thumping them.' Of course, a whole day later, the steam has nearly always gone out of the situation and 'thumping them' seems like a really stupid idea. Another way of relieving your anger and annoyance is to write the perpetrator a letter – then tear it up instead of delivering it; or pretend they are there in the room with you and tell them what you really think of them. Or you could try saying something directly to them such as 'I truly value your friendship/guidance/opinion but you really upset me yesterday. Can we talk about it without getting angry?' With a loved one, ***how about asking for a hug.*** It's a request that only the hardest heart can resist. And it's always worth remembering that laughter is one of the quickest and healthiest ways to dissipate anger and so relieve the associated stress and tiredness.

*** *Take each day as it comes along.* Work on the basis that yesterday has gone and tomorrow never comes. In his book *Love Is Letting Go of Fear*, Jerry Jampolsky reminds us that 'The past is over, it can touch me not. This instant is the only time there is.' It's helpful to affirm these words out loud to yourself when you find that you're fretting over what has gone and over that which is yet to come.

Jerry also shows a lovely cartoon which illustrates a trash can lifted off into the air by a balloon. The man on the ground has loaded the bin with all his guilt, fear and painful experiences and is waving them goodbye! Why not try it for yourself?

*** In everything you do, *consider the other person's point of view* before you jump to the wrong conclusion. They may be feeling unwell or recently bereaved, for example. If you are aware of such possibilities when someone is being bad tempered towards you, it alters your view of the situation and can help to reduce your stress as well as theirs.

*** Smile at people who look as if they are unappreciated. The supermarket check-out operator, the driver of your bus or tram, the postman, the tea lady. *Say 'thank you' and mean it*. You'll feel better and so will they.

*** Don't allow yourself to become a doormat but try to *do something spontaneously for somebody* else every now and then that they would not otherwise benefit from. A smile, a wave, a few flowers, a jar of homemade preserve, collecting someone's shopping for them; take a blanket or a hot meal to someone who you know has to sleep all night in the street. Little things mean a lot, especially to the sad, the elderly, the lonely and the homeless. Being isolated or underprivileged doesn't make them second-class citizens.

*** *Donate clean cast-off clothes and bedding to the Salvation Army.* Your local branch will be listed in the phone book.

*** *Count your blessings* and be grateful for good things. There are plenty of these around even in the most dire of circumstances. It's just that when we are unhappy, we don't see them. When it rains, don't groan about the weather; picture the rejuvenated rivers, the refreshed and refilled reservoirs, dry land being watered and crops soaking up the life-giving liquid. During the darker days of winter, listen to the ground and picture the new shoots of spring pushing their way to the surface. There's an oft-told story of the man who stopped complaining about having no shoes when he met a man with no feet. It's a useful reminder that most of us take our comforts for granted.

*** *Tell yourself every day that you are unique and valuable.* Go on, say it to yourself now. 'I am unique and valuable.' Then write it down on a piece of card and keep it in your purse or pocket.

STRESS BEHIND THE WHEEL

*** According to the Health Promotion Research Trust's three years of research – in conjunction with Aston University, Birmingham, England – driver stress could be driving drivers round the bend. Changing attitudes towards irresponsible driving techniques not only reduces stress levels but can also save lives. The behaviour of other road users, aggressive bumper-jumping, frustration at not being able to overtake, being overtaken, a general dislike of driving itself, needing to keep to a strict time schedule, traffic jams, bad weather conditions and fatigue are all factors which can increase irritation and, consequently, driver stress. Interestingly, too, drivers are more stressed in the evening than in the morning.

*** There is really no excuse for aggressive driving, especially when it achieves nothing positive and risks other people's lives. We have all experienced bad behaviour on the road and, all too often, it is the innocent victim who suffers. The competitive and 'macho' images which occupy the minds of some drivers would be laughable if they weren't so senseless. Few of us are impressed by engine revving dimwits with less brains than a bag of wind who overtake on blind bends and practise the Veteran Car Drivers' signal as they speed by.

*** To reduce your level of driver stress, learn to let them go. They are probably less of a danger way ahead in front of you than they are kissing your rear lights.

*** Make allowances for other people if they drive erratically. They may be learning, they may be lost, they may be elderly, they may be unhappy, worried or sick and consequently not concentrating properly, they may simply be crazy, irresponsible and stupid.

*** Try to be tolerant. What is the point of letting another driver's bad behaviour make you angry or getting all stewed up in a traffic jam you can't do anything about?

*** Make contingency plans in case you get lost. Have the telephone number and address of your destination with you. If you ask directions, repeat them back and jot them down. A few moments of planning can save hours of frustration.

*** Enjoy your car's cassette recorder, CD player or radio. Good music can soothe many a stressful situation.

*** Try to leave other problems behind you. Worrying about work or home will distract you from the task in hand. Don't drive at all if you have just had an argument with someone. Slamming out and roaring off at top speed is a waste of tyre tread and a waste of energy — whether it's gas/petrol, diesel or adrenalin! Calm down first.

*** Don't overtake unless you really need to and have the space to do so safely. Think about how often you have seen a car which shot past you ten miles back, stuck at the next set of traffic lights.

*** Don't sit in the middle lane of the free-way/motorway oblivious to all around you. Lane hogs are a dangerous nuisance. Inside lanes on motorways are often empty of traffic just because lazy drivers can't be bothered to use them.

*** Be more considerate towards drivers of large vehicles. Think about the size and crushing ability of a twenty tonner. Would you like to reverse it, park it, load it, unload it or manoeuvre it around in any way at all?

*** Don't drive for long periods of time without taking a break. Stop, rest, stretch, have something to eat and drink, go to the washroom, freshen up — then go back behind the wheel.

*** Be mindful of the needs of others who may be less mobile than you are. Don't park in spaces reserved for disabled drivers unless you have the documentation which allows you to do so. Such action causes immeasurable stress and dis-stress to people who really do need to park there. It can cause you stress too. Fines and clamps are being used more and more often now to deter un-authorized parking.

*** Don't make promises to arrive at a precise

time if your journey is a long one. Traffic problems can build up unexpectedly.

*** Eat properly, especially at breakfast time. Accidents are more likely if you missed a meal; low blood glucose levels can affect your powers of concentration.

DON'T BE SUFFOCATED BY STRESS

1. When stress strikes, stop banging your head on the wall for a moment and ask yourself if what is happening is worth worrying about. Go on, do it. Is this particular problem going to still be a problem in a hundred years' time? In the case of arguments, most are likely to be forgotten in a day or two, a week at the most. Even the effects of those traumas and distressing events which never seem to go away are unlikely to be hastened by worry. The potential for stress occurring in the first place will be much reduced if you don't overreact and don't anticipate trouble.

2. See the stressor as a plus point in your life, as opposed to a negative one. Become actively involved in what is happening (the only way you can make a difference) instead of seething on the sidelines. Taking control is one of the best ways of dealing with negative stress.

3. See stress as a positive opportunity for change. Look back at traumas which have occurred in the past and you'll almost always discover that something good came out of the experience.

4. Don't go into self-reproach mode about something that didn't go as well as it might have done. You'd be surprised at how much we can learn from stressful situations.

5. Use the tips in this chapter to help control your body's response to stress.

6. Give your body the nourishment and care it needs to protect your system against the ravages of stress attack.

*** If stress is a significant problem in your life, you may also like to read specific books on the subject. Those which I found most helpful are detailed on page 339. But remember, to deal effectively with negative stress in your life, you have to *want* to change things. Taking the view that a situation is hopeless, that change isn't possible, that you have no control – is not going to improve matters. Finding ways to reduce stress levels doesn't necessarily mean a completely different lifestyle; it's often the minutest of modifications which make the biggest impact. A small match can light a large fire!

SOURCES OF REFERENCE:

~ Mitka M. Patients Seeing Doctors for Job Stress Relief. *AMA News* 1991;6(17):16

~ Walker M. The Therapeutic Power of Color – Part I. *Townsend Letter for Doctors*, December 1991 pp 958–63

~ Walker M. The Therapeutic Power of Color – Part II. *Townsend Letter for Doctors*, January 1992 pp 26–30

~ Shedding Light on Seasonal Affective Disorder. *Tufts University Diet and Nutrition Letter* 1994;12(1):1–2

~ Lighting Up Sad Lives. Article in *Sunday Times Magazine*, 24 January 1988

~ *Light, Colour and the Environment*, by Faber Birren, Van Nostrand-Reinhold, 1983

~ Newell, Guy, Stress and Cancer – The Interactions of Mind and Body. *Primary Care in Cancer*, May 1991;29–31

3

Colourful Energy

'The purest and most thoughtful minds are those which love colour the most.'

John Ruskin (1819–1900)
The Stones of Venice

Colour is part of our everyday language. We talk about 'seeing red', being 'in a black mood', 'green with envy', 'blue with cold', 'purple with rage' or 'in the pink'. To overcome a fit of the 'blues', we may decide to recite some 'purple prose' or to 'paint the town red'. We might have a 'red letter day' or see the world through 'rose-coloured spectacles'. By using these phrases, we are making a sub-conscious acknowledgement that colour can, in some way, affect our lives. Even so, colour choice usually remains limited to the occasional porings over paint and wall-paper, the new coat, the car or the curtains. Few of us ever consider colour in terms of how it might influence our health, our mood or our vitality. But it would appear that colour may, indeed, affect the way we feel.

Unfortunately, the amount of research which has been carried out into colour therapy and colour healing is still relatively limited. For some – and especially for the scientist who believes nothing without incontrovertible verification – unproven accounts and testimonial evidence will not be enough.

Sourpuss Henry Ford (he of the car), who referred to a great many things in life as 'bunk', would probably not have given any credence to this idea, either. He was the one who said 'You can have any colour as long as it's black.'

Whatever your view, there is no getting away from the fact that colour says a lot about us as individuals. For reasons which are perfectly understandable, most of us prefer to hole up behind what we see as cautious colours, too nervous to come out from behind the mask of safety. Some people will read 'bright' as brassy or tawdry and view 'dull' as discreet and reserved. But constant use of lifeless colour can also reveal feelings of dreariness, exhaustion, a lack of self-esteem and a 'what's the point' kind of attitude.

Right or not and like it or not, we are judged by our mode of dress. The colours – and the styles – we choose will almost certainly influence the attitude of other people towards us. If it is true that we receive what we reflect, then our colour choice is also likely to have a profound effect upon the way we feel about ourselves.

PEOPLE WATCHING

Next time you are waiting for a train, walking in the street or the subway or standing in a queue, indulge in a bit of 'people watching'. It is an interesting and enlightening pastime.

To begin with, notice how so many people slouch with their heads bowed. Their body language tells us that they feel as if the weight of the world is on their shoulders. Their co-ordination is poor and they often bump into other people, unaware of their surroundings and wrapped up in their personal problems. They look worn and weary. Are they smiling or laughing? Not likely.

Then, look at the colour of their clothing. Forget high fashion. That's not what I mean. People don't usually go to the supermarket or the metro in their Ralph Lauren or Yves St Laurent. No. In some warmer climes and, perhaps, on the beach, brighter colours are given an airing, people laugh and shout and look as though they are positively enjoying themselves. But in most places, grubby grey, creased cream, baggy brown, boring beige, shapeless navy and unbrushed black predominate below sad and sorrowful faces. In general, our clothing reflects our mood and our mood reflects in our clothing.

You may think that this is OK, that we have a lot to be gloomy about. Recession, slump, war, famine, retrenchment and redundancy, taxes, rising prices, rising crime, cuts in public spending, the latest episode of *Prisoner Cell Block H*; it's enough to make anyone feel grey and tired – if you let it get you down, that is!

Discussing colours at this point may seem trite and insignificant but taking a serious look at the colour in your life can be a catalyst for personal change.

> A person who, in general, reacts freely and agreeably to colors – any and all – is likely to have a responsive personality and to be keenly interested in if not well oriented towards the world at large. [A] less enthusiastic neighbor may be of solemn countenance and glum disposition.
>
> Faber Birren
> *Light, Colour and Environment*

SMILE

Ever noticed how attitudes alter when people smile instead of frown?

They become more positive, not so easily depressed by the daily round of bad news.

Colours can 'smile' or 'frown' at you, too. Look at someone directly and they may look away; smile at them and they usually smile back. A smile, like any other strong facial expression, is a kind of proclamation – in this case that you are friendly and approachable. We can also make a similar statement with the colours we choose to wear.

Laughter, smiles and colours have something else fundamental in common as well.

They are all infectious!

And yet, most people seem reluctant to alter the status quo. They may complain bitterly and constantly ('I hate my hips,' 'My bum's too big' or 'My neck is too short') but then continue to wear shapes and colours which broadcast the problem as publicly as a newspaper headline. I have often heard people exclaim that they 'can't wear green' or 'would never buy blue' only to find they look stunning in those colours. Don't be too ready to assume a colour is wrong for you until you have tried it in all its varying shades.

If people don't like themselves or lack self-esteem, they are far more likely to be stressed and lethargic. In truth, they may have a perfectly acceptable anatomy but the shape and colour of their clothing could be 'accentuating the negative' rather than the positive! Unfortunately, we rarely see ourselves as others see us – and hardly ever from the back!

One day last winter, I stood waiting for a tube train at Paddington in London. There was a delay (surprise, surprise) and I took the opportunity to 'people watch'. The platforms became more and more crowded as the waiting time increased and soon there was little room to move. Out of the hundreds of commuters crammed together like sardines in a can, I could see only one bright colour; well, two, actually. A cheerful green dress on the other side of the tracks and my own cerise pink jacket. Everyone else blended together in a kind of grey suit soup.

If I caught anyone's eye during my reconnoitring, they immediately turned away or looked down – except the lady in green who smiled! Interestingly, I have since learned that green is the colour for open hearts but grey (unless accompanied by other colours) can hold people back from expressing themselves. It saddened me to realize that there were probably several hundred potentially cheerful personalities on that platform who, almost without exception, looked tired, unhappy and, frankly, not very well. A colour consultant would have had a field day.

THE SPICE OF LIFE

Colour is, of course, a matter of personal preference and it can be counter-productive to push someone into wearing a colour which they simply don't like. However, the world might be a brighter place if everyone added a little richness and diversity to their clothing. After all, variety is supposed to be the spice of life!

I'm not suggesting that everyone who is currently kitted out in anything less than sky blue pink should suddenly turn up in sequinned socks and a Technicolor dreamcoat but rather that they dip an experimental toe into coloured waters. Try a brighter shirt under the grey suit, a slightly snazzier scarf, a jaunty tie, some bolder jewellery or even a hat! Being a slave to fashion (once the fashionable thing to be) is no longer seen as necessary. Don't be afraid to be noticed. With today's myriad designs – as the song says – anything goes.

WHAT COLOUR AM I?

I tend to wear bright colours. Jade green, royal blue, purple and the aforementioned cerise are real favourites and are often mixed with white. If I wear quieter cream, taupe, grey or black, I usually add a strong, clear colour, a scarf with vivid hues, costume jewellery or accessories which make a bit of a statement. When I was in Australia in March, I was given the 'Loud Bag Award' by some colleagues who took a shine to the cavernous pink and green holdall I used instead of a briefcase! I enjoyed the fact that they noticed; we all enjoyed laughing about it!

That's me, *now* and it says a lot about how I feel – *now*. Not trashy or tasteless, I hope – but happy, harmonious and, above all, colourful.

I wasn't always into brighter clothing. I was born with a naturally pale (and that's an understatement!) complexion, brownish eyes and fine, flyaway reddish brown hair. Natural it might have been, confidence boosting it was not. Because of my 'brown' colouring, I was encouraged to wear . . . er . . . brown. Sort of er . . . earthy looking, I guess. Good camouflage had I been into ornithology or army manoeuvres, not so wonderful for an uncertain and insecure teenager with a flat chest, a large waist and not an ounce of confidence. Arms like a monkey and a back of giraffe proportions meant that blouses never tucked into the skirt and sleeves ended at the elbow.

When tights (pantihose is a much more sensible description) hit these shores, I could wear them only if I walked with knees bent. They were never long enough! Suspenders provided little respite and were desperately uncomfortable because the dangly bits didn't reach the nylon tops; stockings were always too short and were always 'pinging' away from their support system. Once, I remember with pain and embarrassment, the couplings disconnected loudly and vigorously when I stood to attention in the quiet moment at the cinema which used to fall between the end of the film credits and the beginning of the National Anthem! The situation was not improved in any way by my companions, who fell unsympathetically into a snorting, giggling heap alongside me as I tried in vain to look as if nothing had happened. As we crowded out of the building (in those days, nobody budged until the loyal royal tune sounded the last note), the stockings worked their way slowly to my ankles, accompanied by more helpless laughter.

You will have guessed by now that my forays into fashion were less than successful. I felt gauche, gawky, graceless and dull. I cringe when I see photographs of the time but my defence is that, like so many other people, I didn't realize things could be any different.

When the opportunity came, years later, to take an image consultancy training course, something told me I should go for it. Off I went to the airport in my brown clothes with my brown bag and my brown outlook.

It was the experience of a lifetime! I learned not just about colour but shape and style, fabric, skin care, make-up and accessories. Five thousand ways to tie a scarf was fascinating; how to lengthen the legs, hide the hips and make willows from pears was a breeze – but 'How colours can affect our health' seemed to be the favourite topic of conversation with most of us.

Students were encouraged to spend their leisure time out of doors 'people watching' and putting forward suggestions as to how passers-by could be lifted from their obvious melancholy! I spent many a happy hour with new friends in the street cafés of downtown Amsterdam doing 'distance make-overs' on Dutch pedestrians. Quite a few willing souls allowed themselves to be persuaded to college classes for closer inspection. As a result of simple colourful changes, many a butterfly was seen to emerge from a drab chrysalis.

I returned to England a different person. Laugh if you will (if you haven't uttered even one little giggle by this time, I've failed dismally, anyway) but my husband didn't recognize me when I came off the plane. My brown trappings were in the suitcase and I was wearing a purple jacket over a white shirt with a green skirt.

I've loved the colour purple since childhood but never had the courage to wear it. I've read too often that it was associated with solemnity. It never made me feel solemn, quite the opposite in fact. To satisfy those early cravings, I painted the odd wall here and there instead; much to the chagrin of a succession of landladies! Too much purple can, apparently, convey eccentricity (me, eccentric? how dare you!) but mixed with complementary colours, it can be uplifting.

Wearing the right colours now, I FEEL BETTER. I have a different perspective and a new kind of ENERGY!

BROWN IS BEAUTIFUL, TOO

I'm not saying brown is a terrible colour. On some people all shades of brown and its relations can look stunning. One of my dearest friends has a wardrobe full of earthy colours which suit her beautifully, the browns contrasting with orange, yellow, tan, cream, green and turquoise.

Even though her clothes are inexpensive, she always gives the impression that she has just stepped out of a glossy magazine and if she wasn't so genuine and gentle, you might hate her for it! Like the colour brown, she is dependable, steady and conscientious.

She also has tremendous energy.

The really interesting thing is that she looks as tired and as ill at ease in as many of my colour choices as I do in hers.

COLOUR YOU FEELING BETTER

Mention the use of colour and the first thing that comes to most people's minds is the system made famous by Carole Jackson and *Colour Me Beautiful*. The philosophy is based on categorizing the best colours for any individual by assessing hair colour, eye colour and skin tone. Hundreds of different hues are grouped into four basic units which, for ease of reference, are called, rather confusingly, 'seasons'. Whilst each unit or season has its own batch of basic colours, some colours also overlap from one 'season' to another. An interesting point is that solid colours are more likely to achieve better results than lots of multicoloured patterns.

Greens, blues and reds are found throughout but, usually, in different tones or shades of the basic colour. For example, a red for one person could be an orangey red with a yellow base. For someone else, red will mean a pinky red which borders on the blue side of the spectrum. Have you noticed how, for example, you can look and feel terrific in a deep royal blue but tired and terrible in a petrol blue? Or gorgeous in emerald green but ghastly in olive or lime? Or vice versa? The blue is blue and the green is green; it is the subtle differences in depth which make a colour fabulous on you or better on the dog.

ABOUT FACE

One of the greatest *cosmetic* achievements of colour analysis is the effect colour has on the face. Wearing the right choices in clothing can minimize lines and shadows, smooth the complexion and give warmth to the skin tone. The wrong choices are instantly recognizable as those which echo a pale, sallow complexion and accentuate or create circles under the eyes. If you look good, it follows that you feel good. Feeling good usually equates with vibrance and energy!

I can give you a classic example of this. One of my most expensive purchasing errors was made many moons ago when I happened upon a gorgeous ski jacket. Second mortgages were arranged! My alert – as always – husband hated it from the moment I put it on because it was, he said, totally the wrong colour. He was right. It created dark circles under my eyes and made me look terribly ill. It has been consigned, sadly but of necessity, to my 'jobs outside the house in the winter' jacket. Later on, I replaced it with a much less expensive jade green equivalent which looks and feels fantastic.

The success of colour consultancy has encouraged millions of women – and a not inconsiderable number of men – around the world to re-think their wardrobes, update their make-up and re-assess their self-image. And wisely so. At the very least, image counselling – if done properly and professionally – can save you a fortune in gaffes and blunders. No-one gets it right every time but there is a limit to the number of mistakes one can afford to make. The shade which doesn't quite match, the suit or skirt which always feel 'wrong', the impulse purchase which *really would* look better (all together now in chorus, please) . . . *on the dog*!

I have seen lots of less than confident people come out of their shells with a new radiance following colour analysis. If you have never seen it done, grab the opportunity. The results can be sensational. They can also be money-saving in other ways. Many people imagine that the first thing they have to do after 'having their colours done' is to go home, chuck everything out of the wardrobe and start (expensively) all over again. Not necessarily so – unless, of course, that's what you want – and can afford to do it. A gifted consultant will be able to advise clients on how to mix the right colours with the not-so-helpful ones you can't afford to part with and still achieve a dazzling outcome. For example, those black trousers or that grey blouse will look even more terrific if co-ordinated with brighter contrasts. Items which you never thought suited you and have been hanging sadly in the wardrobe for ages will, suddenly, come into their own with a little professional help.

COLOURFUL COCKUPS

Unfortunately, I have also seen some appalling errors made by allegedly talented colour consultants which have left the client looking more pale and wan than they did before they made the appointment. The answer here is to go by the recommendation of people who have been for 'treatment' and who look wonderful after the event. I would recommend a colour coding consultation to anyone who feels down in the dumps, has an important project ahead of them, needs guidance on style and shape, is recovering from illness or is making a new start. Anyone who grouches that it would be a waste of time is probably related to Henry Ford!

JUST FOR FUN

Whether you decide to 'have your colours done' or not, why not invest an hour or two in a wardrobe makeover? Take everything – including accessories – out of your wardrobe. Put to one side any items that you haven't worn for the past two years. If you can't afford to give them to the local charity shop, a second-hand clothes shop will make offers on good quality, used but clean, clothing. The usual arrangement is that the shop takes the clothes on sale or return for a period of, say, six weeks. If they sell them, you will be paid a percentage of the sale price which you can accept as cash or put towards a new outfit.

You'll know immediately whether the shop is worth using or not, by the layout, the attitude and the smell! (Shops which take not-so-clean clothes always smell ghastly whereas a good outlet should be indistinguishable from a regular store.) Good outlets also move with the times, so don't be offended if they refuse items which are clearly past their sell-by date!

SECOND-HAND ROSE?

Some people will baulk at buying and wearing clothing which has been worn by someone else – but it is worth remembering that the system is hardly any different from hiring an outfit. Even brand new garments can be shop-soiled and have probably been tried on by other bodies before yours. If you do buy anything via this route, add to your investment by having the item cleaned anyway. The benefits of second-hand shopping are that you can save an absolute fortune and, with diligent sleuthing, can pick up designer labels at bargain prices.

When you have discarded, one way or another, the items you no longer need, take a serious look at what is left. Wash or dry clean anything that you want to keep but which is not looking its best. Give an old favourite a new look by changing the buttons. If you are handy with a needle and thread, give blouses and shirts a new lease of life by renewing the collars – perhaps with a contrasting material. If not, a few enquiries will find a seamstress in most towns and villages.

Ask yourself if the colours, shapes and styles you have decided to hang on to are really right for you. If the answer is yes, that's great. But don't be afraid to be discriminating. Are you better in an 'A' line or a straight skirt? Should you wear trousers with, or without, turn-ups? Do shirt collars suit you better than scoop necks – or vice versa? Are the hemlines too high or too low – or are they uneven? Those who are well-endowed in the hip department should check that the hemlines don't dip at the front and skim the beam at the back. What do *you* look like in the rear view mirror?

If you go in for separates, how many of the tops and bottoms will mix and match? In other words, how many 'new' outfits can you create from existing stock? (This is fun to do anyway but even easier and more productive if you have had a colour analysis.) Ask a reliable and honest friend to be there with you during this exercise and tell her you'll be glad of a constructive critique. Reciprocate by helping with her wardrobe. You may find a few items to swap.

If space permits, put winter clothes in a different area from summer ones. You'll see them with renewed interest next season if they have been out of sight for a few months.

Clearing, sorting and tidying in this way is believed to be helpful psychologically too, especially if you are feeling run down, exhausted or depressed. A change, they say, is as good as a rest; so is a good clear out!

LIVING WITH COLOUR

In our homes, too, colour choice is an individual thing. In one house that we moved to some years ago, the previous owner had a penchant for pink – unfortunately not the nicest shade of pink and not just in small amounts but *absolutely everywhere*. Pink is one of those choices which can be great in splashes and drops and especially cheering in clothing but very tiring when daubed in great dollops all over the house. One room was so overpoweringly depressing and nauseating that neither Ralph nor I could live in it until that ghastly colour scheme had been eradicated. Now it is a fresh and sunny area of cream and white, contrasted with dark wood furniture, and is our favourite sitting, talking and relaxing room. And we did it ourselves; well, actually, we did get a modicum of professional help – my mother – who made a fabulous job of painting the doors and the ceiling! Never had a lesson in her life but is the *crème de la crème* of decorators and a rag-roller *par excellence*!

When you are feeling down, painting a wall or two can be extremely therapeutic. After all, it could be the existing colour of the room which is making you feel depressed. For example, overdoing the bright reds, oranges or yellows may not be helpful if you are already hyper- and over-anxious. Being completely bathed in blue is not a good idea if you are depressed and feel the cold easily. If you learn a little about colour, however, you will soon know which tones and shades go best with which.

Even if you are definitely not a do-it-yourselfer and turn pale at the thought of filler, undercoat and anaglypta, almost everyone has the wit to paint one wall. I recommend this 'therapy' wholeheartedly to the severely fed up. Sorting through the paint cards can be a bit like turning the pages of a holiday brochure, something to look forward to. Painting a wall could hardly be considered expensive and, you never know, the results you achieve might give you the incentive to go on and do more!

Decorating can be stressful if you look upon every job as a huge project but not everyone can afford the services of a professional. I have overcome this problem to a great extent by calling in the expert only for the more difficult tasks such as unreachable ceilings, arduous stair wells or wallpapers with a will of their own.

Apart from these, I paint on a 'bit at a time' basis, when I *feel* like it. A wall, a door frame, a windowsill. Why knacker yourself trying to do the whole house at once? What does it matter if it takes a bit longer? There can be great satisfaction in being able to say 'I did that.' Don't be daunted. Too many people back away from something with an 'I could never do that' attitude. How do you know you can't unless you've tried? There are lots of inexpensive and really helpful books and leaflets on home decoration available. Colour your life a little and you could feel a lot better.

COLOUR AT WORK

Slightly more difficult at the office, however! Someone might just say something if you suddenly turn up at work with planks, dustsheets, brushes and tins. But the dreariest area can be brightened and made more inviting with ornaments, pictures, postcards, fresh flowers and pot plants (which are also good for helping to reduce pollution). Personalizing your workspace with the right colours is a definite must if you are suffering from fatigue and lack of energy, if you are stressed at work or have not been feeling well.

HOW DO WE SEE COLOUR?

The eye sees colour through a layer of light-sensitive receptors in the retina called rods and cones, aptly named because of their shape. When light falls on the receptors it is absorbed by chemicals which then break up and send electrical impulses to the brain, enabling us to identify darkness, light and colour. The rods pick up on the two extremes of the spectrum, black and white, and contain the pigment *rhodopsin* which helps us to see in the dark. The cones produce other pigmented chemicals which are sensitive to red, green and blue.

Colour blindness happens when one or more cones are missing or damaged in some way, the most common type of disorder being the inability to distinguish between red and green and the most serious when someone is able to view the world only in a kind of monochrome. Night blindness can occur when there is a deficiency of Vitamin A needed to make rhodopsin, the pigment in the rods.

This is a simplified version of the way colour and light sensitivity is explained in physiology textbooks. What it doesn't explain is how living creatures who do not have human eyesight or people who are blind can, in many cases, also distinguish colour. The answer may lie in the fact that colour gives off vibrations and that light has the ability to penetrate the body not just via the eyes but also through the skin!

LIVING ENERGY

A famous experiment carried out in the early 1980s demonstrated that amoebae, the most basic of life forms, actually showed changes in their molecular structure when exposed to different colours; blue made the molecules 'open up' whilst red caused them to pack more tightly together. No eyes, no rods and no cones – just vibrations.

Researchers have discovered that blood pressure can be raised by red and lowered by blue, in the sighted as well as in the visually handicapped. By learning how to sense the rates of vibration, blind people can 'see' colours. There is a now well-known story of a Russian woman who taught herself to differentiate between one colour and another by holding her hands over them and recognizing the varying vibrations. Some people are also able to 'feel' the heat or the coolness of colours.

Put simply, colour is light which is broken down into different wavelengths, each colour being determined by the type of light it reflects or absorbs.

When light passes through a prism, it is 'split' into the colours of the rainbow, appearing as red, orange, yellow, green, blue, indigo and violet. Another uncomplicated way of understanding the existence of colour is to describe it as the vibratory rays which move – at different speeds – between black and white. The speed of the vibration and the length of the ray will determine the colour produced.

Red – at one end of the rainbow – has the longest wave-length and the slowest vibration; violet – at the other end – has the shortest wavelength and the fastest vibration. When light hits an object that absorbs all the colours of the spectrum except one, that is the colour we will be able to see, the one which 'reflects back'. It could therefore be said that objects have no fixed colour of their own but are determined by the level of light which is reflected from their surface. The intensity of a particular colour is decided by the intensity of the reflection.

If you're wondering about transparency, see-through objects are that way because they can transmit all colours equally and reflect little or nothing back to the eye.

Here endeth the science lesson!

COLOUR AND YOUR HEALTH

Colour is more than decoration. It can quieten your anxiety or quicken you into action. It can irritate or placate, calm or excite and lift or depress. Colour can also aggravate fatigue or elevate and restore our energy. And it can help to heal.

It is said that one of the reasons the Aztec Indians painted their bodies different colours was to overcome different ailments, a practice still recommended by some healers today. In ancient Egypt, temples were positioned so that the sunlight which was then broken up into pris-matic colours could be used for healing. Therapeutic sunbathing and the bathing of the sick in areas of special colour is believed to have been practised in Ancient

Greece, Rome, Babylon and Assyria (now Iraq) and Palestine.

Wearing the right colours is important not just for the persona we project to the outside world but for our health too. Believe it or not, colour and light can have a direct effect upon body chemistry. Ultraviolet, for instance, is believed to have anti-bacterial properties, is used in some parts of the world as a treatment for psoriasis and, as most people are aware, is an important factor in the production of Vitamin D. Light has been shown to increase circulation, prevent anaemia, reduce the work done by the kidneys and so assist in detoxification. Light certainly affects hormonal activity and is believed to be one of the most important factors in controlling bodily functions.

Choosing the right colours can make us feel cheerful, positive and confident. The wrong colours not only inflict gloom and despondency but also make us feel less than fit. Someone else's colours can have as beneficial or deleterious an effect on you, the onlooker, as it can on the wearer.

NOTHING TO WEAR?

Different days can call for different colours, depending upon your mood, level of energy and fitness. Notice how an outfit worn one day can feel fabulous and, yet, on another, not seem right at all. Choosing colour is personal and yet is more than merely individual preference; it can also be determined, it would seem, by instinct and need – and may alter with age.

WHAT TO CHOOSE

It's a fact of life that any kind of excess can lead to danger; colour is no exception. Every colour requires moderation and balance. Too much of any one colour can be disturbing and destabilizing. Even a colour that you like very much won't be a favourite for long if you are staring at it all the time. Choosing a combination of complementary colours which suit both your personality and your personal colouring will provide equilibrium, variety and interest.

CONVINCING EVIDENCE

During my research into colour and energy, I found a great deal of fascinating evidence that colour can indeed affect our lives. There is already a mass of data proving the value of colour in many different situations. As studies into the subject become more detailed and sophisticated, I believe that we shall find colour to be more akin to our health than anyone, thus far, could have imagined.

Colour is sometimes used by psychologists as an indicator of personality traits; results can be revealing, informative and, for some, uncannily accurate. The following insight into the effects of colour has been collected and collated from many different sources and references. It is, due to limited space, a general view only; guidelines to have fun with rather than hard and fast rules to live by. But if you have an energy problem, are stressed, anxious or depressed, understanding the effects of colour could be a brilliant beginning.

RED

Those who favour bright red are often fast thinking, out-going, extrovert types who have an appetite for success and are happy with their own company.

Red is sometimes viewed as an aggressive colour. Indeed, sodium vapour street lighting belongs to the red spectrum and has been blamed for an increase in street crime. However, red also signifies strength and can be helpful if you are lacking vitality (although not if you are the type who tires easily). It may also help to warm a chilled body and improve circulation. It isn't necessary for the whole outfit to be red, just part of it. Socks, for instance (with or without sequins!), a scarf or a shirt. No-one expects you to turn up in head to toe red although wearing red underwear is supposed to improve your sex life!

Colours from the orange/red spectrum are also associated with hunger and food; one reason why they turn up so frequently in the decor of fast food outlets! It seems that warmer, louder colours may stimulate the nerves linked to the appetite centre in the brain! Colour therapists advise that dieters who have problems with bingeing and cravings should avoid red, yellow and orange. Don't wear them, don't eat in restaurants which use them, don't paint any part of your house or workplace with them and don't even eat off plates with red or orange patterns. Where restaurants and canteens have changed to quieter colour schemes, snack sales have fallen and those on diets are reported to have lost weight.

Red is not recommended for anyone with high blood pressure as experiments have shown it can increase it.

If you decide on red, don't overdo it. Too much can lead to aggression, restlessness and irritability. Balance it with light grey, white, blue/green or green. Brighter reds which lean towards orange seem to suit those with fairer hair. If your natural colouring is dark, you may be more comfortable in the softer shades, still related to red but with less orange or yellow in their base. For example, crimson, cerise, deep pink, magenta, maroon or burgundy, all of which can be stimulating and uplifting and are great colours for 'getting things done'.

ORANGE

Orange seems to suit the fun-loving socializer and, like the people who favour it, can assert an anti-depressive effect on those around them. It is also associated with youth, vigour, curiosity and restlessness. As with red, orange in small amounts can be cheering but too much hard orange can be overwhelming and tiring.

Interestingly, it is not considered a suitable colour for those in authority as it is said to diminish responsibility. Better alternatives may be peach, apricot and coral which complement well with cooler partners, blue or violet. Oranges and tans are not usually good colours for people with naturally dark hair or dark eyes.

YELLOW

We associate yellow with sunlight and with sunny personalities. Yellow is energizing too and can help to reduce stress. It is also the colour for happiness, creativity and a thirst for knowledge. Those who like yellow are supposed to be mentally alert and clear thinking, sometimes shy and often have an interest in philosophy. Said to be good for loners and high-minded thinkers! Like red and orange, yellow offers far more benefits when utilized in small amounts. On the negative side, too much harsh yellow can be overpowering and even nauseating. Yellow, of course, is also the colour of cowardice and custard.

A splash of bright yellow can look wonderful on the fair haired but for dark haired people, lemon yellow is a quieter alternative and balances naturally and well with lavender, mauve and violet.

GREEN

Green is an 'even' colour in the middle of the rainbow spectrum and is all about amicability, amity and peace. Likewise, lovers of green are said to be balancing. It is no coincidence that green is the colour for conservation of the environment, signifying the tranquillity of the country-side and harmony with nature. It is also the colour of compromise. 'Greens' can, however, be anxious people, always worrying about events outside their control and may be naïve and easily put upon by others.

Unfortunately, green has long been associated with the 'Little People' and so is regarded, rather stupidly in my view, as a superstitious colour. How, for example, do those who are superstitious about green cope with green fields, green trees and green vegetables? The 'green room' so familiar of television studios is supposed to convey conviviality and hospitality but few of them seem to be painted green these days. The right amount of green certainly helps to reduce stress levels and the brighter greens are energizing. Its balancing colour is purple and, together in an outfit, they look stunning!

TURQUOISE AND JADE

These related colours fall between green and blue and have been linked with stability, courtesy and charm but a cool and detached exterior. The semi-precious turquoise stone is used in crystal healing to create a protective barrier around the wearer. Fusspots are supposed to favour blue/green! (Oh dear, I like that one too!) They are also the colours of the sea.

Turquoise is said to be valuable in boosting the immunity and so may be the colour for bedwear in hospital and during convalescence. Turquoise is also believed to be helpful when giving lectures or taking examinations because it calms nerves and helps the absorption of instruction and the conveying of knowledge. Blue/greens and turquoise fare well with purple and lilac. Turquoise is also balancing for brown, an often untried but attractive mix. Blue/green is said to be good with red but, in this case, the choice of shade and tone is important if harsh results are to be avoided.

BLUE

Like a summer sky, blue is an open colour which makes

others around you feel comfortable; it is calming in stressful situations and is the colour associated with inspiration. If you have an important meeting or event to attend, adding blue to your outfit can help to settle those butterflies in the pit of your stomach.

Blue has shown itself to be calming in other ways, too. Where mercury vapour street lighting (which belongs to the blue spectrum) has replaced the red-based sodium lighting, crime rates have dropped. If you have an excitable personality or are needing to quieten an over-active mind, soft and soothing blue can help bring peace and serenity.

'The blues' have always indicated sadness and depression so would not be recommended for anyone feeling down; too much may be a sign that you prefer to ignore the world around you and hide away, in which case a splash of opposite orange provides uplifting balance.

PURPLE

Purple is a proud colour and may be dismissed because of its association with positions of authority, religious robes and grand ceremonials. Too much of it can certainly create heaviness but, in moderation, it can be an exhilarating addition to any wardrobe. Purple people (nice alliteration that) are said to be artistic, witty and sensitive (there, now, that's definitely me) but also impatient and unconventional (whoops!).

Purple complements well with the blue/greens, jade and turquoise. On dark-haired people, it also has particular impact when worn with white. If you are fair or blonde, lilac or paler violet may be a better choice.

VIOLET

Violet is good for balance and concentration but, like all colours, best in small doses. Overdoing it can convey aloofness. Lavender types are often impeccably dressed, gracious and refined but detached. They don't like involving themselves in other people's problems and, it is said, would never dream of getting their hands dirty!

Violet and its related colours, lilac, lavender, mauve and amethyst, are calming, soothing, purifying and can be helpful in relieving the devastation of despair and bereavement. Most interestingly, many therapists find similar healing qualities in the amethyst crystal and in lavender essential oil.

If you wear any of the softer purples, balance them with lemon yellow or one of the blue/greens.

BROWN

Brown can make you feel safe and secure and is the colour often chosen by solid and reliable personalities. A conscientious colour associated with work and, of course, the salt of the earth. Excessive amounts of brown, especially if you already have brown hair and brown eyes, may indicate a fear of flamboyance; brown is easy to hide behind if you resist change. If you really favour brown, try variations of shade such as mushroom or taupe but beware of beige and mustard which can be very draining. Turquoise, cream and powder blue are good contrasts for brown colouring and brown clothing. If you are lighter haired, then try apricot or peach for distinction.

GREY/GRAY

English grey (or American gray) can be either drop-dead gorgeous or downright gloomy, depending upon how it is handled. Overdone, grey can mean lack of excitement, unswerving dedication to duty and fear of smiling. Grey people hardly ever let down their hair and would never throw their hat at a tram (old Northern expression). Greys prefer a quiet social life but may be workaholics around the office. Hence the epidemic of grey city business suits?

Lots of dark grey can be far too heavy and tiring so, if you like grey, go for the lighter shades and mix them with brighter colours. The great advantage of pale grey is that it goes well with almost any other colour but can be especially attractive when combined with red, deep pink, white or purple.

BLACK

Not really a colour but easier to refer to as such, black is the respectful choice for funerals and sadness. Although I defer to those who choose it for solemn occasions, I hope that no-one wears black to my wake.

I think it is a great shame that black is also becoming

the standard uniform of the young. Black leggings, black leather, black accessories, black boots! Big blocks of black are gloomy, depressing and overpowering. A totally black outfit can indicate a suppressed personality, unexpressed anger and difficulty dealing with authority.

Worn well, however, black can be elegant and distinguished. On dark-haired wearers it balances beautifully with white but may not be so attractive on anyone with naturally fair hair. Try blending your black with cream, pink, pale blue or the lighter greens – or, if you are unsure about black, keep it just for accessories such as briefcase, handbag or shoes.

COLOUR, AURA AND THE CHAKRAS

So far, we have talked mostly about the physical use of colour, colour choice and preference, and about how light is reflected or absorbed. Most of us have, at one time or another, felt the effect of colour on our mood even though we might not have realized it then or understood quite why it happened.

We may also have had the experience of meeting someone who made us feel particularly happy and energized and another who may have drained us and made us feel unnerved or unsettled in some inexplicable way.

Almost everyone has surely been affected by the 'vibes', the vibrations, which are given off by others. This 'cloak of energy' which surrounds someone's physical presence is referred to as the 'aura'.

To a clairvoyant, the aura or energy field around the human body is seen as a mixture of moving colours and has been described as a coloured vapour or shield. The colours – and their tones or shades within the aura – will indicate to the clairvoyant the areas of harmony or disharmony (health or dis-ease) within the physical body. Even healers who are not clairvoyant and who cannot 'see' colour are able, in many cases, to pick up a sensation of lightness or darkness about someone's personality through their own hands. I remember one spiritual healer in particular who could identify pain on someone else's body because those areas appeared to the healer to be dark grey. It is said that animals, who often display very accurate intuitive skills about people, use the aura to determine whether a particular visitor is a threat or a friend.

Many colour healers use therapeutic colour to replenish the body via energy centres within the system called 'chakras'. Each of the chakras is allied to a particular area of the physical body, an endocrine (hormonal) gland and, also, to a particular colour and characteristic:

Crown of the Head & Pineal Gland	Violet	Philosophy/ Spirituality
Forehead, Third Eye & Pituitary Gland	Indigo	Clairvoyance
Throat & Thyroid	Blue	Intelligence/ Expression
Sternum	Turquoise	Truth/ Teaching
Heart & Thymus Gland	Green	Compassion/ Understanding
Solar Plexus, Stomach & Pancreas	Yellow	Feeling

continued

Sacral Spine, Reproductive Organs	Orange	Digestion/ Colon/ Relationships
Base of Spine, Adrenals & Kidneys also Sex Organs	Red	Sexual Energy/ Security/ Activity

Working with the chakras and with colour healing can help to 'reload' and restore the body's energy reserves. It can also be a valuable learning tool and an interesting new way of looking at disease, health and the connection between mind, body and spirit.

There are many variations and different aspects of colour healing; I have only touched on the subject here for interest's sake and would urge anyone who is considering colour healing to seek out an experienced practitioner. The etheric body is sensitive and easily unbalanced. Don't dabble without professional guidance.

A FINAL THOUGHT

How sad it is that we choose to discriminate against a person's skin colour when, really, all we are doing is showing prejudice against the speed and density of particular rays of light! Puts racial disharmony into perspective, don't you think?

SOURCES OF REFERENCE:

~ *Colour and the Human Response* by Faber Birren, Van Nostrand-Reinhold.

~ *Light, Colour and the Environment* by Faber Birren, Van Nostrand-Reinhold, 1983.

~ *Healing Through Colour* by Theo Gimbel, C.W. Daniel.

~ *Colour Me Beautiful* by Carole Jackson, Piatkus Books.

~ *Frontiers of Health* by Dr Christine R. Page, C.W. Daniel.

~ *Why the World Isn't Grey* by Hazel Rossotti, Pelican.

~ *The Luscher Colour Test* edited by Ian Scott, Pan Books.

~ *What Colour Are You?* by Annie Wilson and Lilla Bek, Aquarian Press.

~ *The Healing Power of Colour* by Betty Wood, Aquarian Press.

4

Don't Abuse Your Sleep Switch

'Fatigue is the shortest way to Equality and Fraternity – and, in the end, Liberty will surrender to Sleep.'

Friedrich Nietzsche (1844–1900)
German philosopher

Many members of the animal kingdom are synchronized by the rising and setting of the sun. My cat, Sylvester, is completely tuned into this. He crashes out into the deepest of sleeps when darkness falls, snoring loudly, but leaps into live wire action as soon as daylight chinks in. This is fine in the winter months but not so great in the summer. He has difficulty understanding that we are not as keen as he is to investigate the precincts at daybreak or join in the dawn chorus at 4 a.m! I've had other cats who have been just the opposite – insistent on a midnight prowl and un-rousable during the day. Others still have enjoyed a series of naps throughout the twenty-four hours – usually fairly lengthy ones! – with short periods of wakefulness in between. The point is that animals are canny. They know that to remain awake and alert they must also take sleep and rest.

People are not so sensible. In line with our burning desire – an almost suicidal tendency, in fact – to take everything to extremes, people have long wanted to conquer both day *and* night. Now that we have invented electricity (it's not so easy to master the dark with candles alone), we have created 'controlled time', inventing shift work, alarm clocks and a twenty-four hour society. Our modern culture is one which encourages us to neglect the need for sleep.

The *natural* inclination for humans is to sleep during the night and wake up during the daytime, an activity which is commanded by the charismatic sounding suprachiasmatic nucleus – our 'biological clock'. Located in the hypothalamus, an important communication centre in the brain, the 'clock' can recognize what is happening in the outside world via the eyes. It 'sees' daylight and gently nudges us into wakefulness; dusk approaches and it sends snooze signals to encourage us to cease our activity and to rest. It is perfectly natural for us to want to sleep longer in the winter and rise earlier on bright sunny days.

The hypothalamus and its team orchestrate the daily, circadian rhythms of our bodies and the secretion of the hormone, melatonin, responsible for helping us to sleep. Also under its direction are body temperature and alertness. The brain's lowest ebb and the body's lowest temperature both occur before dawn when we are supposed to be tucked up in bed but, for a variety of reasons, often are not. Blood glucose levels are also at their lowest at this hour, hypoglycaemia being a common perpetrator of inertia, slowed reactions, hallucinations and nightmares (see page 162). Almost everyone has experienced the hobgoblins and gremlins of melancholia and coldness which can disturb the wee small hours.

Like the children in the book *The Land of Far Beyond*, it is easy for our imaginings to take on a more sinister character during the hours of darkness – and all because our brains are tired and our bodies chilled. In the story, the guardians, Sleep and Rest, guide a group of tired travellers past the Dragons of Fatigue who, at night, are bestial and bellowing fire. The children are, understandably, terrified. In the morning, the well-rested youngsters can't believe how small and quiet the 'dragons' seem. When they ask how this can be, Sleep explains to them that, at night, we can't see things properly and our troubles always seem far more worrying and distressing. When Sleep and Rest have cared for us, we see things more clearly and for what they really are; in other words, not nearly as complicated or as scary as we first thought and much easier to resolve. The illustration (by Horace Knowles) of the benevolent and beautiful Sleep quietening the dragons and protecting the children from danger is one well worth looking at and remembering when night fears come out to prowl.

CATCH AS CATCH CAN?

There have been many discussions and disagreements over the years as to whether or not it is possible to 'catch up' on lost sleep. But the latest research would seem to suggest that we can. It isn't always possible to crash out for the regulation stretch – indeed, not everyone seems to need eight hours. Some require more and some much less. But what is important is that we take regular sleep and, also, that we recognize our own individual need.

DREAM TIME

Different phases of sleep occur throughout the night in ninety-minute cycles. The REM (rapid eye movement) phase is our dreaming time. Although researchers do not fully understand the function of dreams, it is believed that they serve as a kind of emotional dumping ground or sorting office for information which hasn't been filed during the day. The novelist William Golding explained it well when he said 'Sleep is when all the unsorted stuff comes flying out as from a dustbin upset in a high wind'! People who are deprived of REM sleep can suffer depression, fatigue, restlessness, irritability and even anger and aggression. When returned to normal sleep cycles, subjects spend longer in the REM phase, making up for lost time; confirmation that 'catching up' on sleep is necessary.

DRUG DILEMMA

Sleeping pills seem to offer a simple answer to sleep problems but beware. Short-term use of drug medication during a particularly difficult time is unlikely to have any long term detrimental effect but permanent usage should be questioned. Drugs which act on the central nervous system (i.e. certain sedatives, antidepressants, 'recreational' drugs and painkillers) can suppress REM sleep and disturb the balance and regularity of sleep cycles. One of the reasons why those on nightly sleeping pills often have vivid dream recall is because REM sleep has been suppressed throughout the night until the drug begins to wear off towards morning. The body then tries to make up for lost dreaming sleep. Because the dreams are condensed and concentrated into the interval just before waking, they are remembered more clearly and intensely.

A similar rebound reaction occurs when drugs are withdrawn.

Inadequate sleep and the consequent disruption to the natural body rhythm and biological clock are insidious. Fatigue, poor performance, lack of co-ordination and poor concentration creep up on you, unnoticed. If they continue unchecked, exhaustion sets in, health deteriorates and accidents become much more likely.

DANGEROUS BUSINESS

The inquiries into major disasters around the world – nuclear accidents, tragedies at sea, rail crashes, near misses in the air – found that many of them occurred during the night or the early hours of the morning and were set in motion not just by human 'error' but by human fatigue. The darkest hour of many a catastrophe has, indeed, occurred just before the dawn.

A WORLD THAT NEVER SLEEPS

Before the sun has set in one part of the world, it is rising in another but, because technology has enhanced the level of instant communication and increased the speed of transport, it has become impossible to switch off either of the hemispheres when night falls. Even while some of us sleep, others around us are awake, keeping the globe moving at an ever-increasing pace.

There is no doubt, however, that without sleep, the body cannot repair and recharge. Health and wellbeing are at serious risk, stressful situations become more difficult to cope with, energy levels take a downturn and, guess what, we can't sleep.

We may feel that we have too many people relying on us and that taking time off to rest and reset our natural body rhythms is impossible. ('What will people think of me?'; 'How will they manage?') But as Dr Christine Page points out so graphically in her beautiful book *Frontiers of Health*, if we refuse to step off the treadmill voluntarily, circumstances may take the upper hand. In other words, if we fall ill due to stress, fatigue and lack of sleep, the enforced bed rest can provide a time to reflect on life and to discover that no-one is indispensable. As Dr Page gently reminds us, 'Nothing happens by chance.' How much better, then, to take preventive measures.

The English dramatist, Thomas Dekker recognized the connection over *400 years ago* when he wrote 'Sleep is that golden chaine that ties health and our bodies together.' Modern scientific research confirms that sleep deprivation, nutritional deficiencies, stress and over-exercising can all have adverse effects upon immunity to illness. The fact that we tend towards too much stress, too little sleep, not eating properly and, perhaps, an obsession with physical fitness, doesn't bode well for our long-term future health.

THE BEGINNING OF HEALTH IS SLEEP (Old Irish proverb)

The only truly effective way to overcome lack of sleep is to sleep. If we are to maintain the energy to cope with the society we have created for ourselves, we have to learn that we cannot continue to work without rest or remain well or wakeful without sleep.

I'M A MORNING PERSON

People may say they work best at a particular time of day, whether it be morning, noon or night, perhaps a sign that we are intuitively aware of our own personal 'body clock'. The actual time of our birth could be a factor here, being the shock moment when we arrived in the world and the clock started 'ticking'. Although it doesn't apply in every case, it is surprising how many people who were born in the morning feel that they function more efficiently earlier in the day. Those born late at night are often the ones who are wide awake at midnight. I met someone recently who told me that she was born at midday and feels, instinctively, that this is her best 'performance time'.

OLDER AND WISER

As people age, they often find that they go to bed later or waken earlier in the morning. 'I don't need as much sleep as I used to,' you might hear someone say; and it does seem to follow that sleep requirements reduce as the years advance. On the other hand, older people, especially after retirement, have more time on their hands and may have greater opportunities for catnaps during the daytime. Add up all the sleep they are taking in a twenty-four-hour period and, for quite a few, they are sleeping for the same length of time as always — only in shorter, more frequent bursts. Those of us who are still on the gravy train should learn from this experience.

JUST FIVE MINUTES MORE

Regular naps or rests are known to improve performance and help reduce energy loss. ENERGY, ENERGY, ENERGY. Remember? About 85 per cent of mammals accumulate sleep through an aggregate of brief naps per day; but, for humans, napping is not recommended as a replacement for fully rested sleep, rather as an additional recharge or as a strategy to get you through a bad patch. Carry on for too long without proper sleep and you will find it more and more difficult to function.

There is also a condition called 'light sleeper syndrome'. This has nothing to do with railway tracks but is a type of 'false insomnia'. Many people complain of not sleeping ('I lie awake *all* night') when, in fact, they do sleep quite well. Because their level of sleep is not as deep as normal, they imagine they are awake for hours on end. Some people who dream vividly may dream that they are awake and so have the mistaken idea that they didn't sleep well.

SHIFTING AROUND

Research has shown that shift workers who alternate regularly between day and night duty suffer a type of permanent jet lag because of the disturbance to their natural sleep rhythm as well as inadequate exposure to natural light. As a result, their health profiles are not as good, they have poor concentration, a greater number of accidents and, not surprisingly, suffer from ongoing fatigue. Those who are on fixed and steady day *or* night shifts appear to be able to adjust their body clocks to cope. They do not seem to suffer the same level of health damage or deprivation because they sleep properly during their time off. Gaining access to natural light during at least some waking hours is an important factor in sleep regulation, too.

NO BETTER THING UNDER THE SUN

Although we hear much about the 'leisure society' which is supposed to be spending more time out of doors, the fear of overexposure to ultra violet radiation (promoted with equal fervour by media, medics and manufacturers of sun tan lotion) has driven many people to cover or coat every square inch of bare flesh with fabric or fluid. There we go again; excesses and extremes. Either we brown to a crisp or we hide. No compromise. Mad dogs, Englishmen and idiots go out in the *midday* sun but there is no reason why we should avoid the gentler sun of early morning and late afternoon.

Unless we suffer from the condition of photosensitivity (abnormal skin reactions which occur on exposure to sunlight), a little sun-seeking is vital to our health and wellbeing and especially essential to anyone who suffers from insomnia. Inadequate exposure to sunlight may, in turn, slow down natural melatonin production, disturbing our body clock and natural sleep rhythm. Even a peek outside on a grey overcast day can be healthful. Perhaps we should heed the words of the 19th-century English poet Matthew Arnold: 'It is so small a thing, to have enjoyed the sun, to have lived light in the spring.'

WHAT HOPE OF ANSWER?

Plenty! Investigators have come up with some useful recommendations for improving sleep patterns which, in their turn, can help to reduce stress and increase energy.

*** Before giving in to drug medication, try the relaxation and breathing exercises which begin on page 240. Deep breathing is known to be calming and encourage sound sleep. It really does make a difference so don't neglect this first resort.

*** Try to avoid bell and buzzer alarms. Do without if possible or use a radio alarm which starts the day with music. If you need a cacophonic stimulus to break your sleep cycle, it could mean that you have not taken all the sleep you need.

*** Try going to bed five or ten minutes earlier each evening until you are retiring an hour earlier than previously.

As you relax, waiting for sleep, say out loud to yourself 'I will wake up at . . .' By stating a time which is a few minutes before your usual alarm call, you may find that you need only to set the alarm on rare occasions (for a vitally important appointment, for example). Many people say that they wake up only seconds before the alarm would sound, enabling them to turn it off before that blast of adrenalin jolts them into space. Another adjustment of the body clock, perhaps?

*** During the day, even on overcast days during the winter months, try to spend some time outside. Natural daylight can be up to thirty times more intense than the brightest artificial light and our biological clocks need daylight to trigger the melatonin which helps us sleep. If you suffer from insomnia or depression 'natural daylight' bulbs can be helpful but they are not a substitute for real outside daylight.

*** Invest in a little bit of power-napping; it can do wonders for your power-dressing. In other words, taking naps during the day, switching off for anything between five and forty winks, can recharge your system and switch on your energy.

*** Invest in some relaxation tapes or CDs or listen to classical music or a radio play. A unit which switches off automatically is a real investment for the despairing insomniac. You'll be surprised how frequently you miss the end of a programme!

*** If an attack of insomnia hits you, don't lie there 'mythering'. Mind chatter is not only intrusive, it can be destructive too. Be active; get up and do something. Read, make yourself a warm drink, listen to the radio, do some deep breathing exercises. On the rare occasions that I wake during the night, I listen to the BBC World Service, some light classical music or a relaxation cassette. Sleep comes when it's ready. I love to listen to audio books but spend a good deal of time rewinding the tapes next morning!

*** If you have a late night or an earlier than usual start, make up for it by taking more rest and sleep in the following forty-eight hours.

*** A cup of coffee or tea can help to give you an emergency 'lift' if you are forced to keep awake, but don't rely on uppers to keep you up. It's well known that too much caffeine, especially if consumed during the evening, can lead to attacks of insomnia.

*** During the day, try to drink more filtered or mineral water and less in the way of stimulants. It's worth knowing that office air conditioning can remove up to one full litre of water from the body in only a few hours!

*** Check out your diet. According to naturopath Dr Ross Trattler, sleep problems have been linked to deficiency of B vitamins, too many refined, sweetened foods, sensitivity to food additives, excess alcohol or a diet which is too high in salt. A consultation with a qualified therapist who is familiar with nutritional treatments may pay far more dividends than a quick fix sleeping tablet.

*** Don't eat a heavy meal late at night. If your digestion is being forced to work overtime, you will find it more difficult to doze off.

*** But don't go to bed on an empty stomach either. Waking up with night sweats could be a sign of 'night starvation' or nocturnal hypoglycaemia (low blood sugar). A light snack taken an hour before bedtime can help you to sleep.

*** Invest in regular sessions of reflexology. Regular treatment does appear to reduce anxiety and increase the likelihood of a good night's sleep.

*** 'Restless legs' syndrome (twitchy, sometimes painful limbs) is a common perpetrator of insomnia. Although it can affect anyone, restless legs seem to be more common in women and in the elderly. Avoiding tea and coffee during the evening has been shown to reduce discomfort. Also, taking a low dose B Complex and 300iu of Vitamin E with breakfast and a multi-*mineral* (not multivitamin) complex with supper has reduced symptoms in some sufferers and relieved the condition completely in others. However, not all supplements provide the same degree of quality and so not all makes will be effective. If you take multi*vitamins*, swallow them with breakfast or lunch. Used at night they may stimulate you into wakefulness. More details on pages 315 and 328–330.

*** Painful and neglected feet can throw your whole body out of balance, causing headaches, restless legs, neck tension and a variety of other symptoms which may keep you awake. Devote a few minutes each day to your feet whether you decide to have reflexology treatment or not. Keep toenails in trim. If nail cutting is difficult for you, see a chiropodist. Massage (unperfumed) body lotion into your feet after your daily bath or shower. Add two drops of lavender oil to the body lotion before applying. You'll find more information in the chapter on Stress which begins on page 9.

*** A warm (not hot) bath before bed can help to induce sleep. Add five drops of lavender oil to the bath water and, also, put a couple of drops on a tissue under your pillow.

** See a chiropractor. Spinal misalignment appears to be a neglected but common factor in insomniacs. A short course of treatment followed by a six-monthly check-up is a real health investment.

*** Try to isolate the reasons for your insomnia. Are you worrying unnecessarily about something? Is there a problem which would be resolved if only you could discuss it with someone? Are you feeling unwell but afraid to talk to your medical adviser? Have you fallen out with a colleague, a friend, a loved one? And is it preying on your mind? Having the courage and resolve to take action can be the very thing which releases the tension. Talking it out with yourself, out loud if possible, is a good way to straighten a distorted perspective.

*** Being afraid of the dark can be stressful and sleep-disturbing. It is a common problem and nothing to be embarrassed about. Do you know someone, an elderly person or a child perhaps, who is sleeping badly and afraid to ask for help. Leaving a light on outside the bedroom can be comforting and is a good security measure. Do you have a telephone connected in the bedroom in case of night-time emergencies? In our homes, we should be able to relax and sleep peacefully and without concern. Is your house as secure as it could be? Ask your local Crime Prevention Officer to call and advise you on additional security measures. The service is free in most countries. The physical security of extra locks for doors and windows can help to give emotional security. Make sure, however, that you have a planned escape route in case of fire. Fit smoke alarms now and contact your local Fire Service who will give free advice on fire safety. Numbers are in the phone book.

*** If insomnia is a real problem and you can't work out what is causing you to sleep badly or to lie awake all night, ask your GP for a health check. Make it a priority. There are a number of conditions which can cause or aggravate insomnia (and sap your energy too). These include thyroid problems, menopausal symptoms, heavy metal poisoning, nutrient deficiency, allergies, stress and, of course, pain.

*** Hypnosis has helped some insomniacs. If you decide to seek professional help, take the time to find a qualified practitioner. Self-hypnosis is also valuable as is Autogenics. For further information, see Further Reading on page 343, and How To Find a Practitioner on pages 352–353.

*** Are you sleeping in a safe place? Have you considered the possibility that geopathic stress may be affecting your property and, in particular, your bedroom? In our modern technological society, we are surrounded by weak electromagnetic fields which emanate from airports, early warning radar, electricity pylons and substations, electrical equipment, radio transmitters and a host of other high-tech apparatus. The experts who study geostress believe that this kind of equipment could be harmful if the electro-magnetic wavelengths being given off become distorted and then pass through our houses or offices. Equipment in the home is also surrounded by electrical and magnetic fields which can emanate low frequency rays.

Until relatively recently, exposure was thought to be harmless but new research has suggested that health may, after all, be detrimentally affected. According to the journal *What Doctors Don't Tell You*, considerable evidence now shows that living near to relatively low level magnetic fields given off by mains electricity cables can raise the chances of childhood leukaemia by at least three times.

The book, *Are You Sleeping in a Safe Place* by Rolf Gordon explains how the distortion of the earth's natural rays can detrimentally affect our health and well-being and the importance of removing harmful pollution from our sleeping areas. For further information on this see Further Reading on page 342.

You should also ask *What Doctors Don't Tell You* (details in Further Reading on page 340) for their special report on Power Lines, Volume 5, No. 3, which contains a great deal of self-help information, including how to arrange for your property to be tested for EMFs. Use only recognized consultants and don't fork out for expensive equipment unless it is recommended by bona fide experts.

Check out the chapter on Energy and the Environment (page 125) for more information.

*** Transcendental Meditation (TM) is a simple, natural technique which, if practised daily, can induce a state of deep rest in both mind and body. Research shows that TM is valuable in the treatment of stress-related conditions, insomnia, migraine, blood pressure problems, asthma, angina and drug dependency – with no adverse side effects. A study in Canada indicated a 36 per cent reduction in medical expenditure in those who used TM regularly. For further information on TM and details of training centres in your part of the country, contact the TM National Communications Office. Details are on page 357. Freephone 0800 269 303 or 01695 51213. Books and tapes are also available. In other parts of the world, TM practitioners and classes are usually listed under 'Transcendental Meditation' in your telephone directory.

*** For those who – genuinely – don't sleep so well, there are many sleep remedies worth trying. In one study of nine individuals, aged between 68 and

80, it was found that a 2mg capsule of melatonin before bed enabled them to fall asleep more quickly and sleep for longer. The same medication has been used successfully on people with jetlag. If you have explored every avenue and are no further forward, talk to your doctor about the possibility of a short course of melatonin. Limited use at low doses may be sufficient to realign an out-of-kilter body clock.
*** The herb Valerian has long been used as a sleep preparation and there are many brands on the market. They are not, however, generally available on prescription. Valerian does not behave in the knockout way of some sleeping drugs but rather quietens the mind and slows the body down in readiness for sleep. Products sometimes contain a mixture of other plants too. For example, Passiflora (Passion Flower) acts as a mild tranquillizer; Scullcap may help to reduce muscle pain and cramps whilst Hops are calming. None of these botanicals is believed to be addictive.

Regular use of low doses is worth trying if you have a problem sleeping or are going through a particularly stressful or anxious time. In one study which tested the effects of Valerian on sleep patterns, the subjects taking part reported better quality sleep with no side effects and no nightmares – two common problems with prescription sleeping drugs.
*** Try a Hop Pillow. An old-time cure for insomnia was to put hops into a piece of muslin under the

pillow. Nowadays, Hop Pillows come packed for the purpose.

*** Prescription sleeping drugs should be treated with extreme caution and taken only as a last resort. Short-term use at low doses may be suggested as a crisis measure to get you through a bad patch but permanent use should be considered only in extreme cases. If drugs are recommended to you, make sure that you discuss dependency and side effects with your doctor. If information is not forthcoming, think about changing your GP or seeking a second opinion.

** If you find yourself folding with fatigue during the day but have no opportunity to 'drop off' even for a few minutes, here are ten emergency energy boosters:

1. Get up and move around
2. Stretch
3. Yawn
4. Seek out some fresh air
5. Take some deep breaths
6. Eat something
7. Inhale the aroma of a stimulating essential oil such as Lemongrass and Eucalyptus or Peppermint and Melissa
8. Drink a glass of water
9. Massage gently around your ear lobes
10. Turn on some music

5

Leaving on a Jet Plane?

'For millions of years our ancestors were ruled by the laws of day and night. Since then we think we've got smart, that we've conquered the night, but in reality that's just an illusion.'

Dr Martin Moore-Ede
Author of The 24 Hour Society

Flying has become an inescapable fact of life; in its vapour trail comes the almost inevitable jetlag. The easiest way to escape jetlag is to stay at home but that means no long haul business trips and no far flung holidays. Avoid flying and you don't get to go anywhere that necessitates crossing seas and oceans – unless you have the time to go by ship/boat/yacht/raft . . . or just happen to be sailing single-handed around the world anyway.

Air travel can be a pleasure or a pain, depending upon how you plan and how fit you are. If your job and your livelihood hinge on frequent flying, then it's probably unavoidable. All the more reason to be prepared.

Unfortunately, in keeping with much of our modern lifestyle, flying is a fairly unnatural thing for humans to be doing. If God had meant us to fly, we would have needed more than wings. Undercarriage, reverse thrust, radar and telepathic radio links spring to mind. It's no use humans flapping their arms about all over the place if they turn up in Boston instead of Brisbane and then can't land without breaking bones. Hang-glider handy in your pocket, is it?

Lots of things about aeroplanes make flying an unhealthy business. High altitude, cabin pressurization, changing time zones, electromagnetic pollution and radiation, low humidity and dehydration, sitting with your knees under your chin for hours on end, sleep deprivation, lack of natural daylight, the 90+ decibel in-cabin noise level, the toxic stew which is laughingly referred to as air-conditioning – all *conspire* to make you *expire* . . .

. . . not to mention the in-cabin 'gassing'.

And you wonder why you feel exhausted?

IT'S A GAS!

On flights to certain countries, the cabin is filled with fumigating anti-bug sprays, usually ejected into the passenger areas before landing. Even domestic flights in some parts of the world are keen on saturating the atmosphere with pesticides, especially where there may be regional proliferations of certain undesirable pests. (Did you say you can think of one or two undesirable pests you *would* like to include? Same thought occurred to me.)

As far as my research can determine, there is no legal requirement for passengers to be advised about gassed flights before boarding which, effectively, means you can't know which ones are fumigated and which ones are not. There is no detectable odour given off by the sprays.

AIR *CONDITIONING?*

In addition, a bad dose of flu or a heavy cold are common

side effects of air travel. If you 'go down with something' after almost every flight, the reasons shouldn't surprise you. Four hundred or so people all sharing the same air is likely to result not only in oxygen starvation but in a cosy exchange of recycled viruses too. According to Diana Fairechild in her book *Jet Smart*, most jetliners provide between 40 per cent and 60 per cent 'fresh' air, the rest of it having been passed by the management, so to speak. Unfortunately, the filtration systems are not designed to filter out infectious bugs so you are powerless to avoid breathing in someone else's germs. Why do you think they strap you to your seat before they blast the back of your neck with cold air?

Unless it is a non-smoking flight, cigarette smoke is an additional toxin to contend with and one of the major contributors to stale air and oxygen deficiency. Even though filtering units deal with some of the fug, it doesn't get it all. Some 'non-smoking' seats are so close to the smoking area that the designation is a joke.

Oxygen levels inside aircraft are, according to Diana Fairechild, less than adequate, unless you are a first class passenger (their area receives better quality air); or can afford to go Concorde, the only plane which provides completely fresh air. During the research for *All Day Energy*, I spoke with senior personnel at Qantas and British Airways and am assured that strenuous efforts are being made to improve fresh air ingress and the quality of air conditioning on all flights.

The inevitable hypoxia (oxygen deficiency) which occurs during flight can lead to shallow breathing, light headedness, physical and mental fatigue, poor co-ordination, impaired judgement and poor memory; if prolonged, nausea, twitchy limbs and headaches may also occur. Flying also disrupts the body's endocrine system (hormones to you and me) which means that menstrual cycles can be thrown off key. Periods may turn up earlier or later or heavier than usual or may be missed altogether. Lack of oxygen also means that carbon dioxide wastes are not expelled as efficiently, the circulation is more sluggish than normal and less nourishment is delivered to the cells.

Important note for nervous flyers: If you are worried about the pilot doing an oxygen-starved wobbly, don't. Flight deck crews receive around ten times the ventilation of the main cabin (that's *fresh* air, not recycled) on the basis that *them as flies the plane needs to be bright-eyed and bushytailed*. Well, we are all very relieved to hear that, aren't we!

UNAVOIDABLE RADIATION

The atmospheric layer which surrounds the earth acts as a safety blanket, blocking out much of the high energy radiation from outer space. The higher we travel away from the earth's surface, the less protection available. The result is an increase in exposure to many types of radiation.

Air density, air pressure and oxygen availability are all reduced at high altitude which is why it becomes necessary to pressurize aircraft cabins. This is done by taking a large volume of low density air, compressing and cooling it and then ducting it into the cabin to keep the pressure at a life sustaining level.

All these factors disrupt the body's cellular harmony, creating an excess of toxic chemical malcontents called free radicals, undesirable and unstable molecules which, through a chain reaction of cell vandalism, can damage tissue and reduce the body's ability to fight infection and repair damage.

Under normal circumstances, the body organizes its own damage limitation exercise by calling on antioxidant vitamins, minerals and free radical bashing enzymes. Unfortunately, it would seem that, in many people, their nutrient reserves are already low because of constant exposure to other hazards at ground level such as stress, environmental pollution and inadequate diet. In the inhuman environment of an aircraft, however, this defence system is put under considerable further strain. It is the resulting loss of cell protection which reduces vitality and increases the likelihood of jetlag.

Researchers have found that one way to help overcome jetlag is to put the protection back into the system in the form of enzyme supplements. Taken just before and during flight, they can go a long way towards reducing the unpleasant symptoms of jetlag. For more information, see page 355.

JUST PLANE SCARED?

If you are a seasoned and confident plane Jane – or Jim – you probably think that the word 'aerophobia' means being frightened of the bubbles in a certain brand of air-filled chocolate. For a few people, however, there is one particularly significant – and very unfunny – source of stress which, inevitably, increases the likelihood of jetlag: fear of flying. And the terror is not always confined to the actual flight.

Freaking out because the taxi is late picking you up or being nervous about finding somewhere to park the car, getting claustrophobic in the lift or lost in the airport building, convinced that you'll miss the plane, losing your luggage or being locked in the aircraft washroom only add to the worry.

It sounds an old cliché but is nevertheless true that flying is, from the arriving safely and in one piece point of view, one of the safest forms of transport. Crossing the street or going out in the car are far more dangerous. But because we walk and drive on terra firma, we have a sense of control over our activities and so f-e-e-l safer. A dread of heights isn't likely to be a problem on the ground unless, of course, we are unavoidably detained at the top of Centrepoint, the Chrysler Building or British Telecom Tower!

At thirty or forty thousand feet, however, someone else is doing the driving. For the duration of the flight, you have *no* control over your situation. You have no choice but to put your trust in the pilot.

I think I was probably a touch nervous the first time I went up in a plane; fixated on the life jacket and oxygen mask demonstration while the rest of the blasé bunch read their free newspapers. If we have a prang, I thought smugly, I'll be the first down the safety chute because I'm the only one here who remembers where the door is.

Have you ever filled out one of those 'wary canary' quizzes which appear occasionally in magazines? In the questionnaire that I came across most recently, 'the plane goes into a sudden dive but the pilot assures the passengers that all is well.' They wanted to know if I would 'study the safety leaflet' (I looked already) and 'locate the nearest emergency exit' (I watched the demo, remember?), 'listen out for unusual noises in the engines' (I'm suddenly an aircraft engineer?) or – get this – would I 'order a drink and watch the end of the movie'? Who are they trying to kid? I'd call the steward, check the dinner menu and ask if this was some kind of new system for landing the plane more quickly. Piece of cake, as they say in the RAF. Me, afraid of flying, nahhhhhhhhhh!!!!

Someone once told me that even the thought of a 'Fear of Flying' course was enough to send them running for the train station but, joking apart, the airlines do a convincing job. Staying afraid of flying is not only restricting from a geographical point of view, it also leaves a potentially damaging stressor untreated. In these days of fast transport and mass communications, the rest of the world is on everyone's doorstep. It can be a handicap if a suppressed fear or phobia prevents you from seeing any of it.

LEAVING THE JET LAG BEHIND

Helpfully, airlines are now getting the message that reducing, overcoming or preventing jetlag is likely to increase their passenger fan club. Most people have one or more personal tips on how to reduce the effects of lagging; here are some more to add to your list:

1. Sleep. If you can catch some kip during your flying time, then your risk of jetlag will be significantly reduced. Even half an hour to an hour

can make a big difference. Studies carried out with long-haul air crew and other shift workers has demonstrated that even short bursts of 'micro sleep' can improve performance, reduce fatigue and increase energy levels.

The following notes should help you to relax and achieve good quality rest.

2. Plan ahead. During your normal routine, cut down a little on your intake of stimulants i.e. coffee, tea, chocolate, cola, sugar, salt and alcohol.

3. If possible, try to avoid wearing pantihose, stockings or any kind of tight clothing.

4. However tempting it may be to tuck into the on-board booze, don't drink anything alcoholic either immediately before or during the flight.

5. Say no to any orange juice offered to you and opt for bottled water instead. Cartoned and bottled juice can be very acidic and appears to cause headaches, migraine and digestive upsets in some people.

6. Refuse ordinary 'aircraft water' or ice. You never know which country supplied it or what it might contain. Bottled water should be available; if in doubt, take your own. You'll definitely need it. Pressurized cabins are dehydrating to an amazing extent – around half a litre of water an hour from the body during flight is a conservative estimate!

7. As soon as you board the aircraft, set your

watch to 'destination time'. The Captain will usually make an announcement about this soon after take-off. When you arrive, fit in to whatever time that happens to be. If you land in the morning, take things easy but avoid going to bed; stay up, stay dressed and eat at the (new) normal mealtimes. If you arrive at night, follow the tips on bathing (Numbers 9, 18 and 19 in this list) and on relaxation, and go to bed, even if it is only for a few hours. Don't get stressed or worried if you can't sleep. Lying down and resting in a comfortable *darkened* room will still be helpful in resetting your body clock.

8. If you feel lightheaded or are having difficulty breathing during flight, call a member of the cabin crew. If the problem is identified as lack of oxygen, they should be able to supply you with an oxygen mask.

9. Every hour, rub your temples and the soles of your feet with a mixture of lavender and geranium essential oils which, together, are calming and balancing. If you arrive at night, put a few drops of the same oils into a warm bath before going to bed. If you arrive earlier in the day, use juniper with rosemary oil to stimulate, cleanse and help you unwind. Some companies now produce special packs of ready-mixed oils for use during and after the flight but I always prefer to take and mix my own.

Products and Services on page 345 has information on where to find top quality oils.

10. Avoid cigarette smoke, whether it is your own or someone else's. Throughout my life, I have had a serious allergy to cigarette smoke which makes me very sick indeed if I don't give my system additional protection. In aeroplanes, it can be a real problem if my seat is close to the smoking section. If you are a non-smoker and keen to stay that way, book non-smoking flights whenever possible. If you think you may be inflicted with a fug-stirring flight, contact the airline direct (or your travel agent) in advance and book a seat number well away from the smoking area.

It is a well reported fact that smokers are often found to be lacking in Vitamin C – their systems use more of it to counteract the damaging effects of smoking on the body. Less well known is that *second-hand* smoke also causes first-hand vitamin loss. One statistic I came across suggested that 25mg of Vitamin C is used up by every cigarette smoked. Another, reported in the *American Journal of Clinical Nutrition*, shows that smokers have lower levels of Vitamin C in their bodies. Even more worrying is the report from the Stanford Center for Research in Disease Prevention that non-smokers who breathe in other people's smoke can have 'alarmingly low' levels of Vitamin C in their blood. This is what happens: The toxic bonfire spews out pollutants which can damage the cells and increase the risk of heart disease, respiratory disorders and cancer in smokers and non-smokers alike. Vitamin C acts as a scavenger which helps to destroy the dangerous free radical compounds produced by the smoke. If there isn't enough Vitamin C reserve, the risk for serious ill health rises significantly.

Whether you are a smoker or someone who spends any length of time in the company of other smokers, take one gram of a Vitamin C Complex every day and three grams daily when you are flying. (This should be in addition to any other supplements you may be swallowing.) The Products and Services section on page 355 gives details of suppliers.

11. There are now available some specialized supplements for jetlag (made from natural ingredients) which are designed to be taken on the day before the flight and during the flight. I use them with great success on all my long haul flights and have not been troubled at all by any form of jet lag. You'll find further details on page 355.

12. When booking your flight, choose the vegetarian option. Although there are strict rules about hygiene, never forget that the food on your flight (like the water) will usually have come aboard at the previous destination. This

may have been a hot country and one where food-borne diseases and parasites are more likely. Going veggie for the duration reduces the risk of eating foods more susceptible to food poisoning (meat, seafood, etc.). In addition – and according to a senior flight steward – special meals are usually prepared separately and with more attention.

13. Keep warm. If you are being frozen to death by the air conditioning, ask for a blanket.

14. Take a bag of fresh fruit with you for the flight but remember to eat fruit separately from other food to assist digestion.

15. Prevent travel sickness before it starts by avoiding hunger. (This rule applies not only in the air but also on land or at sea.) Sounds strange but it works. Although food is the last thing anyone fancies when their head is already down the toilet, keeping the appetite satisfied maintains a balanced blood glucose level and so reduces the risk of nausea and vomiting. Hypoglycaemia is a common companion to motion sickness.

   Homoeopathic remedies are available which, if taken regularly, may ease the condition – but, honestly, the best way to stay upright is to stay fed. No heavy meals, just light and frequent snacks.

16. Get up during the flight and walk around. Even this low level of movement can help keep

circulation flowing and reduce fatigue.

17. As soon as possible after you arrive, go out into the fresh air and sunlight. Exposing your skin, especially your face, to moderate and sensible levels of sunshine increases production of the hormone melatonin which is known to improve sleep patterns and help balance the body clock. (See chapter on Sleep page 89).

18. Whatever time of day or night you reach your destination, take a bath with the appropriate essential oils. According to Fairechild, this clears the skin of the potentially damaging positive electrical charge which you picked up in the aircraft. If there is no extractor fan, ventilate the bathing area by leaving a window or door open; this allows the chlorine gas, from the tap water, to escape.

19. Brushing the skin before bathing can help to detox the system and swap positively charged ions (which can accumulate during flight) for the healthier negatively charged ones on the skin's surface. Use a skin brush, a loofah or even a rough flannel cloth to stroke the skin firmly, covering all the areas within your reach. However, don't strain to brush the inaccessible parts of your back.

20. The homoeopathic remedies *Arsenicum Album* (Arsen.Alb) and *Natrum muriaticum* (Nat.mur) are useful options for treating the side effects of anti-malaria tablets. The herb Artemisia

Annua is another useful remedy for those who cannot — or choose not to — take anti-malaria medication. However, *be sure to discuss any alternative choices with your GP before you leave home*. See pages 350 and 355 for details of how to obtain homoeopathic remedies and other supplements.

21. Daily garlic supplements are helpful for keeping mosquitoes at bay and are an essential first aid treatment for jippy tummy. It is worth keeping in mind that odour-free garlic products are unlikely to be effective in these circumstances. Put simply, it's the stinky stuff that works but worth it if it saves *you*, your holiday or business trip from disaster. Another tip worth knowing (and these are about the only two situations where I would make this particular recommendation!) is that Pepsi-Cola or Coca-Cola can provide quick and effective emergency relief for food poisoning and for travel sickness. They raise blood sugar, help to balance sodium/potassium levels (which are often disturbed by diarrhoea and vomiting) and assist in the annihilation of bugs in the tum; all useful attributes if you are plagued with nausea, sickness or diarrhoea. In my experience, the Pepsi- or Coca-Cola brands are the most reliable. Local 'own' brands in some countries may be bottled with the very *local* water which upset you in the first place! However, I stress the

words 'emergency use only'! Not an alternative to professional medical advice or treatment.
22. Some airlines run special 'Fear of Flying' courses for aerophobics. In the UK, contact British Airways on 0161 832 7972 for further information about courses in Manchester and London.

In Australia, contact the Australian Women's Pilots Association, 23 Huntingdale Avenue, Miranda, New South Wales 2228. Telephone (02) 522 8455 or (02) 522 8709.

For information about other airlines, contact your travel agent or your nearest airport.

SOURCES OF REFERENCE:

Schectman G et al. Ascorbic Acid Requirements For Smokers – Analysis of a Population Study. *American Journal of Clinical Nutrition* 1991;53:1466–70.

Clemetson C A B. Vitamin C and Multifactorial Disease. *Journal of Orthomolecular Medicine* 1991;6(3&4):161–4.

Caren L D. Effects of Exercise on the Human Immune System: Does Exercise Influence Susceptibility to Infections? *Bioscience* 1991;41(6):410–415.

Castor D. Effects of Sunlight on the Sleep Patterns of The Elderly. *Journal of the American Academy of Physician Assistants* 1991;4(4):321–6.

Shaffer M. Melatonin could help elderly sleep better. Article in *Medical Tribune*, 22/07/93: page 15.

Ayres S, Mihan R. 'Restless legs' syndrome. Response to vitamin E. *Journal of Applied Nutrition* 1973;25:8–15.

Lindahl O, Lindwall L. Double Blind Study of a Valerian Preparation. *Pharmacology, Biochemistry & Behaviour* 1989;32:1065–66.

Notes taken from *Against The Clock* (The 24 Hour Society). Book produced by BBC *Horizon*. Programme transmitted 25/04/94.

Jet Smart by Diana Fairechild, published by Flyana Rhyme Inc., PO Box 300, Makawao, Maui, Hawaii, USA 96768.

Best S. Power lines – the leukaemia link. *What Doctors Don't Tell You* 1994;5(3):1–3.

The Land of Far-Beyond by Enid Blyton, Grafton Books.

Sagan L A. Epidemiological and Laboratory Studies of Power Frequency Electric and Magnetic Fields. *Journal of the American Medical Association* 1992;268(5):625–8.

My thanks to Carl Dransfield in Australia for the additional research notes and information which have been so kindly provided.

I am grateful also to Qantas and to British Airways for their assistance.

6

Energy and the Environment

'Whatever befalls the earth, befalls the children of the earth. We did not weave the web of life, we are merely a strand in it. Whatever we do to the web, we do to ourselves.'

This quote is attributed to Chief Seattle of the Dwamish tribe of the Pacific Northwest taken from the tribal assembly of 1854. This was preparatory to the Indian treaties that surrendered Dwamish land on which the city of Seattle now stands.

We hear and read a great deal about 'the environment' and that monolithic perpetrator of everything that is bad, 'pollution'. But the prophetic words quoted above weren't written about today's pollution problems, they were penned more than 140 years ago. Yet, like that naughty child that refuses to learn by its mistakes, we are still hurling noxious gases and chemicals at the planet. Akin to a boomerang out of control, toxicity has a very nasty habit of rebounding as if from nowhere; rising up to haunt us when we least expect it.

In some parts of the world, people have pooled resources and pulled their ecological act together, restoring devastation and creating new life. But these tend to be single issue campaigns. Elsewhere, particularly where there are larger populations, more intensive agriculture or a greater industrial density, pollution eradication or control has not faired so well.

Almost daily, we are warned about a new threat to our survival; pesticides in pigs or chemicals in clingfilm, toxic tampons or contaminated carrots. Paracetamol screws up the liver. Increases in breast cancer are linked to polychlorinated biphenyls, organophosphates or hydrocarbons, pesticide residues are reported to be present in 29 per cent (a conservative estimate?) of our food supply, wood preservative is blamed for immune disorders and infertility, air pollution for respiratory disease and by-products of the chlorine industry for damage to the nervous system.

Paint fumes can make you feel sick, changing the bed linen can bring on the sneezes and food colourings might give you a migraine. As fast as we wipe out one disease, several more take its place. As fast as we clean up a lake in Africa or save sea birds from yet another oil slick, our farm animals are turning into 'pharm' animals and our farmers are going under from the sheep dip.

The whole kit 'n' kaboodle is enough to give you a thumping headache.

Perhaps the time to really start worrying is when a government 'spokesperson' assures us that there is absolutely no risk!

Obscure acronyms abound but everything will be hunky-dory, apparently, as long as we avoid PVC, MIC, BSE, BST, CJD, CFCs, VOCs, EMFs, PCBs and VDUs. (Difficult, that, since I'm sitting in front of one at this very minute, writing to you.)

Pollution is a tiring business.

There seems to be little doubt that lots of people are affected adversely, to a lesser or greater degree, by many of the so-called 'advances' of modern living. In the years leading from the twentieth to the twenty-first century, there is, at last, acceptance that exposure to 'toxic environmental agents' is affecting our health and our energy.

Almost without exception, the huge number of factors that could be listed under the general heading of 'pollution' have been invented and/or introduced to us pollution-hating humans over the last 100 years; 'state-of-the-art' technology or the seeds of our own destruction – depending upon your viewpoint – but, nevertheless, not really enough time for us to adjust or evolve to the tremendous changes which have taken place.

How many of our ancestors do you think were troubled by:

Vehicle exhaust fumes
Food additives
Pesticides
Chemicals found in tap water
Hydrogenated fats
Instant coffee
Cola
Sugar
The contraceptive pill
Horror movies
Space invader games
Antibiotics
Laxatives
Indigestion remedies
Take-aways
Sleeping pills
Electrical and electronic equipment
VDU screens
Strip lighting
Street lighting
Chemical fertilizers
Herbicides

127

Fungicides
Painkillers
Tranquillizers
Gas heaters
Phenols
Benzene
Trichloroethylene
Formaldehyde
or
Polyvinyl chloride

Had enough? I think so too.

THE BENEFITS OF MODERN TECHNOLOGY

You could suggest that our forefathers might have been glad of the odd antibiotic painkiller, a car or two to get around in or a few pesticides to save their crops from annihilation by the latest coachload of locusts. In small quantities, most pollutants are tolerable and tolerated. It's the larger amounts – and the accumulation and addition of other pollutants to the load – which is causing concern. In other words, it's a question of degrees. Limited or 'protected' exposure (as in, you can't avoid the wretched stuff but you do whatever you can to look after yourself) means that you have a far better chance of keeping fitter for longer.

BUT WHY SHOULD ANY OF THIS AFFECT OUR ENERGY LEVELS?

Primarily, pollutants use up nutrients and place our systems under unacceptable levels of stress. If our bodies are not properly protected by the highest possible level of nourishment, then cells can age more quickly, might not be replaced, could mutate or die.

SOMETHING IN THE AIR?

Energy-lows, especially if they are associated with nausea, travel sickness, headaches or dizziness, have been linked, amongst other things, to an overload of air pollution. Road vehicles and wastes from factories are the most likely source of trouble but vapours can also escape from faulty gas installations, stoves, kitchen ranges or boiler units, blocked flues or clogged chimneys.

DANGER: ELECTRICITY!

The low frequency rays emitted from electrical and electronic equipment can add to the pollution overload. For example, experimental evidence suggests that the magnetic fields produced by AC (alternating current) can produce physiological changes in the human body. AC is the form of current most widely used. To protect ourselves as much as possible from this ever-increasing electromagnetic millstone, we need – firstly – to accept the presence of geopathic stress and – secondly – to understand something of the way in which it can affect human beings. Geopathic stress can occur when natural electromagnetic fields are distorted, i.e. geological structures, natural radiation or underground water, for example. It can also be created by man-made inventions such as radio and television waves, radar signals, electrical and electronic equipment and so on. Humans are bombarded with electromagnetic exposure as never before, much of it unavoidable. However, there are steps which we can take to reduce our risk. Check out the Pollution Protection Points farther on in this chapter.

FOOD OR FAKE

Along with the increase in air pollution – and over a similar time span – a great deal of the food which used to be prepared at home from unadulterated basic ingredients has been replaced by reconstituted, coloured, preserved 'pseudo food' which masquerades, like a wolf in sheep's clothing, as healthful and handsome. Nutrient-deficient junk is hardly likely to help towards pollution protection but does anyone really care? The food manufacturers? The Government? The Health Service? Unfortunately, it is common for those invited to comment or advise on dietary standards to also be in the pay of the very companies who are doing so much to degenerate our food supply. Do we rely too readily on advice given by those who are profiting from the product they are promoting? 'Toxic environmental agent' suddenly takes on a whole new meaning.

Even if the experts are slow to respond, the general public is not. Thankfully, the vast majority of consumers seem to be better informed than the average food manufacturer would wish. I know from my own experiences, especially with patients and students, that interest and concern over such things as convenience foods, irradiation, hydrogenation, additives and pesticides is very real.

OUT OF THE MOUTHS OF BABES . . . ?

I was recently told the story of a seven-year-old girl who spotted the word 'fortified' on a food packet in a supermarket. 'What does *that* mean,' she asked, pointing at the labelling. Before mum could come up with an answer, a sales assistant stacking shelves nearby – and clearly suffering from a severe attack of jaundice – offered: 'Fortified? That's the same as enriched, which basically means that the manufacturer stripped the food of all its taste and goodness during processing and had to add a few vitamins and minerals, colourings and flavourings before they could legally palm it off on a gullible public.'

'I expect that means *we* won't be buying it then,' said the little girl.

ILLNESS ON THE INCREASE?

Can it be a coincidence that, despite improved living conditions and mind-blowing advances in surgical procedures during the same period, nearly everyone can lay claim to their own personal health problem(s)? Almost everybody knows somebody who is affected by cancer or heart disease; allergies and asthma are on the increase; the devastation of AIDS and ME have mushroomed from nowhere and practically everyone you talk to is tired.

Even taking into account such things as increased life span and the practical eradication of infectious diseases such as typhus fever, diphtheria, smallpox and tuberculosis, we seem to be getting sicker instead of fitter.

Ask anyone 'How are you?' and the honest reply would probably be 'Not so great, thanks.'

WHEN RESISTANCE IS LOW, DEFENCES ARE DOWN

Researchers know that over-exposure to toxic pollutants not only damages cells and tissues but also uses up/destroys the very nutrients which we need for protection. Called 'oxidative damage', it can be triggered by an almost countless number of agitators; organophosphates and organochlorine pesticides, vehicle exhaust emissions and cigarette smoke (passive or direct) to name but four. Add a few other pirates such as overexposure to stress, lack of sleep, poor diet, radiation, sugar, food processing, drugs, household chemicals, over-used soil, crop spraying and solvents and you have the beginnings of a health-destroying, energy-sapping cocktail.

DEFENCE CUTS

In small amounts to a well-protected system, the above 'agents' may cause little or no damage. But to an already exhausted individual with reduced defences, the toxic load can become overwhelming. 'Like termites gradually eating away at a house, the rate of damage exceeds the rate of repair,' is how one doctor describes the cumulative effects of pollution.

IMMUNE PROTECTION

Defences can, however, be bolstered. Simple and sensible precautions which cut down the toxic intake are a first step. Encouraging healthy detoxification of accumulated 'debris' is another. A nutrient-dense diet backed up by additional supplements – an important third.

Studies show that people who have low levels of system protection and high exposure to toxicity may not be able to release toxic residues as easily as those who are better nourished and under less pressure from pollution. Researchers believe that this hypersensitivity and chronic toxic exposure (often referred to as 'environmental allergy') may be a trigger for – or even the actual cause of – some of the more serious health problems. Chronic Fatigue Syndrome (aka ME) is a case in point (see pages 193–195).

Unfortunately, modern orthodox treatments do not always have the answer. 'By following current medical protocol, the sick get sicker, quicker;' so says one of the United States' leading experts on environmental medicine, Dr Sherry Rogers. Those who take steps to cut the overload, who have a good diet and a sensible supplement programme may be reducing their risk to both acute illness such as recurring colds and throat infections as well as to long-term degenerative disease.

OK. That's enough gloom and doom for one lifetime. Now let's get positive. Pollution and all its trappings are, to a certain extent, inevitable. Sure, we can campaign, sign petitions, join Greenpeace, support Friends of the Earth, cycle instead of drive, recycle bottles and cans, collect old newspapers for charity and start a compost heap. But what can we do – directly – to help our health, to reduce our risk of illness and, above all, to get rid of this epidemic of exhaustion?

It's no good relying on the food, pharmaceutical and chemical giants or on government; there are those who believe that they don't give diddly squat about your health unless it happens to coincide with making money or collecting votes. At a conference in Sydney, Australia in July 1993 which discussed public health and environmental issues, Professor Charles Kerr from the University of Sydney's Department of Health opened the proceedings with these words:

> How are [the] custodians of our health going about the business of protecting us from chemical hazards in the environment? The short answer is not too well and rather patchily. Governments tend to put the emphasis on economic development rather than get embroiled in endless conflicts over protection of health.

Oddly enough, the more research I undertake, the more positive I become. If nothing else, reading about something which is potentially disastrous increases our awareness and gives us the opportunity to take action.

Professor Kerr again:

It is true that an enormous amount remains to be learnt about toxicity. But there is little point in dwelling on the obvious and, indeed, over the last decade, the environmental mood has been changing towards a more purposeful and positive stance.

I hope that the following tips will help you to collect a few positive pollution-protection points. You'll find more information in the food and supplement sections on pages 257 and 307.

*** Make sure that the vehicle you drive is serviced regularly. Ask that particular attention is paid to the exhaust system, especially if you suspect carbon monoxide may be creeping into the cab.

*** When filling up the tank, try not to inhale too strongly or directly. This is one area where deep breathing is not recommended! The fumes given off by the fuel are just increasing your toxic loading level.

*** Don't pour fuel from a can into a vehicle in an enclosed space – for example, in the garage with the door shut.

*** When hiring or buying a vehicle, ask if it has a 'Recirc' facility; in other words, can the intake of air from outside be shut off and the in-cab air be recirculated? This is useful if you find yourself bumper to fender in a smog-filled city centre, stuck in a traffic jam or being suffocated by a diesel-belcher. Better to breathe your own carbon dioxide for a short while than everyone else's carbon monoxide!

*** If at all possible, choose a vehicle with air conditioning but do remember to leave the window down for a few minutes each time you turn on the air-con. This simple precaution reduces the risk of any bugs which might have set up home inside the system transferring their allegiance to your nose, throat or lungs!

*** Have your central-heating and home air-conditioning systems serviced and your chimneys and flues checked annually. If you are worried, call the engineer now – that means right away!

*** Make sure stoves are properly vented.

*** Check that the flue is open when stoves are in use.

*** Remember that escaping gases don't always give off odour and cannot usually be seen, so that you may not know they are there at all. This makes regular servicing even more vital. One small tip is that a persistently yellow-tipped flame either on the pilot light or main burner can be a sign that undesirable gases are about.

*** Turn on the extractor fan when you are cooking.

*** Don't use a barbecue in an enclosed space. Make sure there is plenty of fresh air circulating around and that fumes can escape.

*** If you are using a mobile space heater, make sure that either a door or window is left open or that an extractor fan is running.

*** Fit heat, gas and smoke sensitive alarms in your home.

*** Ever noticed that, some days, the bathroom smells like a swimming pool? If you are filling the tub or taking a shower, the same ventilation rules apply – this time to allow the chlorine gas to escape.

*** Make sure that any pool you use is properly maintained. Ask how often the pH levels are checked. When chlorine and other chemicals are added, the pH balance is disturbed, making adverse reactions more likely.

*** Always shower thoroughly after a swim. Rinsing with plain water is not always sufficient to remove all the chlorine, so use a body cleanser as well. Don't forget to shampoo and condition your hair too. Avoid ordinary soap, it can cause further skin irritation. Eye drops can be helpful to wash chlorine away from the eyes.

*** Do whatever you can to avoid cigarette smoke. At best, whether taken passively or directly, it can sap your strength, make you *smell* like an old ash tray and *look* like a wrinkled old prune; that means you wrinkle on the inside as well as on the outside! At worst, it is laced with noxious fumes which have the power to kill.

** Talking of noxious fumes, avoid Pavement cafés that are located on busy roads. They may look romantic but just imagine all that grit, grime and gas landing in your *cappuccino*!

*** Try to avoid walking any distance near to a busy road and never take exercise in busy traffic areas.

*** If you bike, wear a smog mask. Useful, too, if you have no choice but to be a pedestrian in a polluted area. Who cares what they look like?

*** If you suspect you might be working in a 'sick' building, i.e. concrete and more concrete, lots of strip lighting, lots of noise, electrical and electronic equipment, etc., then take regular breaks outside in the fresh air, or, at the very least, in a quieter part of the building which is, hopefully, less polluted and more restful. Ten minutes every two hours would be good. It has been estimated that an office worker can waste between 20 per cent and 30 per cent of energy fighting mentally against noise pollution. Staying for too many hours in that kind of environment is bound to be exhausting.

*** Unless you live or work in an area of chronic air pollution, open the windows.

*** Don't wear plastic or rubber-soled shoes at work, particularly if you work with computers. They increase the levels of static electricity.

*** Make sure your VDU has the best quality filter screen available, that you have a footrest if you need one and that your chair is comfortable and at the right height (the seat squab should be sloping slightly forwards and the back of the chair should support your lumbar spine). Check that the lighting is adequate and that you take regular breaks.

Legislation in some areas now requires employers to also provide regular eye tests.

*** Rinse your face and hands regularly throughout the day with fresh clean water and reapply moisturizer suitable for your skin type. The strong electrical charge which is given off by computer terminals can increase the risk of skin blemishes. Rinsing the skin – and taking regular doses of fresh outside air – can change the polarity and 'wash away' the potentially damaging positive ions which encourage bacteria.

*** Eat more fresh fruits, vegetables and salads. Aim for two to three pieces of fresh fruit daily and three or four portions of salad or vegetable foods. These foods are rich in important antioxidant vitamins and minerals and are believed to help lower the risk of cataracts, stroke, heart disease, cancer and other illnesses.

*** When you have control over your food intake, choose organic produce – and free-range eggs and meat – wherever possible. The risks of consuming crop spray residues and drug residues in animal products over time are difficult to assess. However, studies show the organically-grown varieties to be, on average, twice as rich in nutrients as comparable commercially-raised products and 25 to 30 per cent lower in toxic metals such as mercury and lead.

*** Make sure that you wash ALL produce thoroughly before use. Most people will remember to wash vegetable and salad foods but forget about fruits. For example, do you always wash apples, pears and grapes before you sink your teeth in? A thorough swishing and rinsing of fruits and vegetables is good but soaking them can leach out vitamins. Many commercially grown foods are not only sprayed, possibly with pesticides, herbicides and fungicides, but also waxed to improve appearance and shelf life. Sometimes, waxes and fungicides are mixed together. Scrubbing will remove some wax; peeling will dispense with all of it. Unfortunately, however, peeling also means you'll lose a fair amount of fibre. If you are wondering whether to peel or not to peel, the answer is *no* for organic produce but *yes* for waxy non-organic foods such as apples, cucumbers, capsicums (peppers) and tomatoes. If you would have peeled it anyway – bananas, melons, citrus fruits – still make sure to wash it thoroughly first. Skins carry bacteria which will transfer to the produce as you peel it.

It's worth knowing that most stores stock organic potatoes these days. If yours are not organic, then don't use the skins.
*** Locally grown produce may be a better bet than supermarket stock which has been shipped in from long distances. However, avoid buying from roadside stalls. Produce is likely to be contaminated with residues from vehicle exhausts.
*** Filter your water. A good filter jug will cut down considerably on potentially harmful toxins including lead, cadmium, aluminium, nitrates and

chlorine. See page 357 for details of suppliers. Drink plenty of filtered water every day. Bear in mind that some bottled waters can contain more bacteria than tap water.

*** Start each day with a glass of lemon juice and filtered water. This cleansing drink is stimulating and also helpful to the liver and kidneys.

*** Get into the label-reading habit and do what you can to avoid foods which contain artificial additives. Your liver has enough work to do without being forced into dealing with extra unnecessary or undesirable chemicals.

*** Surround yourself – at home and in the workplace – with pollution-hungry plants. There are many varieties which help to reduce pollution in the atmosphere; for example, *Allomena, Dracaena deremensis* (Janet Craig), *Cereus Peruvianus* (the Mexican cactus), *Chrysanthemum, Chlorophytumelatum* (the familiar spider plant), *Philodendron oxycardium* (with the heart-shaped leaves), *Tulbaghia fragrans* (sweet garlic) and the Chinese evergreen *Aglaonema* are useful – as are fresh herbs such as Rosemary, Chives and Mint – grown in pots around the home and office.

Make sure you choose suitable plants for the situation. For example, is the atmosphere dry, cool, warm or moist? Is the room dark with little or no natural light or is there plenty of daylight? Does strong sunlight stream in at certain times of the day? Check with a qualified florist for advice or check out some of the books on the subject in your local bookshop. *The New House Plant Expert* by Dr D.G. Hessayon is an excellent guide on how to look after your house plants. Living greenery can also be soothing and calming, so invest in some plant life if you feel stressed or anxious.

*** Use natural materials wherever possible around the home and office – and for your clothing. Natural wool, cotton, linen and hessian. Choose old wood, old stone and old bricks as building materials. Choose lead-free paints and steer clear of toxic wood preservatives.

*** If you are looking to replace your furniture, avoid the foam-filled stuff. Why not invest in items – second-hand or new – made from natural materials?

*** If you are painting anything or having new carpet or new furnishings fitted, make sure the area is well ventilated. Open the windows.

*** Install ionizers, particularly in your working area. These help to gobble up the undesirable positive ions which accumulate and to recharge the negative ions in the air. Fresh air and sunlight have a similar effect so get outside as much as possible, too, especially if you work all day with electrically-powered equipment.

*** We can't avoid being in close proximity to electrical equipment but, with a little planning and forethought, can keep it to a minimum. It is particularly important to cut down the amount of electrical equipment in your sleeping area. The chapter on Sleep contains more information. Most importantly, contact *What Doctors Don't Tell You* (ask for their Special Report on 'EMFs') who can provide extremely useful information on how to deal with electro-magnetic pollution. Address is in Products and Services – page 340.

*** Locate your television set as far away as possible. Never sit close to it, even when it is switched off. TV sets in bedrooms should be placed around eight feet or more from the bed or, preferably, removed from the bedroom altogether.

*** It's worth knowing that electric blankets can produce their own electromagnetic fields. If you are addicted to your electric blanket, make absolutely certain that it is switched off (at the wall socket) – and preferably unplugged – before you get into bed.

*** Experts recommend that radio alarms, electric clocks, battery packs, tape recorders and CD units should not be placed too close to the bed. It may be less convenient but it's safer. There is another plus point: if you have to get out of bed to turn off the alarm, you are less likely to go back to sleep!

*** Switch switches off and, if possible, unplug at the mains when equipment is not in use. Make good use of copper bracelets. Wear one on your wrist, place another on top of your television set and a third on your bedside table. (See page 349 for Supplier details). Whilst scientific research has now given credibility to the 'old wives' tale' that copper bangles can be helpful to some arthritis sufferers,

my investigations thus far cannot find any solid evidence why they should help people who are affected by low frequency electromagnetic fields. However, there are many individual reports from people whose health has improved as a result and in any event, something so simple is surely worth a try. It's a fascinating fact that the live line linesmen who maintain and repair high voltage pylon cables are safeguarded by special clothing which has copper wire woven into the fabric. The current is then channelled harmlessly around the linesman's body instead of – perilously – through it. Electricity is, indeed, a marvellous servant but a menacing master.
*** Have your microwave oven checked regularly for leakage. The supplier should be able to help you. And if you must use the microwave, don't put salt in the food. Studies carried out at the University of Leeds in Yorkshire, England, suggest that adding salt before cooking may make it more difficult to heat the food evenly and thoroughly. All down to electrical currents and the movement of molecules apparently. Worth following unless or until proven otherwise; it comes from the same department which blew the whistle on the seriousness of mad cow disease when the Government was telling us the opposite!
*** If you think you may have asbestos materials or lead pipes in your home, seek expert advice from your local council or water authority.
*** Ask the water company to test your tap water.

I saw a patient recently whose test revealed 4000 times too much aluminium and 800 times too much iron! Now the situation has been remedied, she is feeling much better, thank you!

*** If radon gas is a problem in your area, contact your local council or health authority for help. Radon testing is available in the UK. See Products and Services on page 347.

*** Use glass, earthenware, enamel and stainless steel in your kitchen. Avoid plastic wherever possible. The chemicals used in their manufacture can leach into the food or fluid that they contain.

*** Choose environmentally-friendly cleaning products. See pages 346–348 for further information.

*** Avoid clingfilm wrap if you can – certainly don't use it on fatty food.

*** Use a vacuum cleaner which is recommended for its filter system. In other words, one that traps the majority of dust in a 'small particle retention system' rather than chucking it out the other end and back around the room. Change the dust bag and renew or clean the filters frequently.

*** Vacuum the mattress every time you change the sheets. Vacuum, also, around and under the bed.

*** If possible, open the windows daily – and especially when you are cleaning.

*** Try to choose bedding made from natural fibres and always change bed linen frequently. Don't forget to pay attention to quilts and blankets too. Shake them in the fresh air and wash them regularly.

*** Consider investing in special mattress and pillow covers which reduce the proliferation of house-dust mite. However, these work well on new bedding but may not be effective if fitted to older mattresses. Dry clean agencies will clean feather pillows which, once aired, can then be covered with this new material.

*** If you need to have clothes or furnishings cleaned, hang them in a well-ventilated area, without their polythene covers, before putting them away. Don't store dry cleaned items in the bedroom. If you have your duvet dry cleaned, make sure it is properly aired away from the sleeping area before putting it back on the bed.

*** Dampness encourages house-dust mites so make sure beds are aired daily. Don't have bedroom temperatures too low or have heaters turned up too high; both can encourage dampness and/or condensation. Fifteen degrees Celsius is the temperature recommended by the National Bed Federation. If you keep plants in your bedroom, choose ones which prefer a dry atmosphere. Greenery which needs lots of water will add to the relative humidity in the room.

*** If you think this is all over-the-top, consider these revolting statistics: A well-fed dustmite has a life span of around six months and will produce twenty dung pellets a day. The waste products it leaves behind have become one of the most common and most serious sources of allergy in the modern

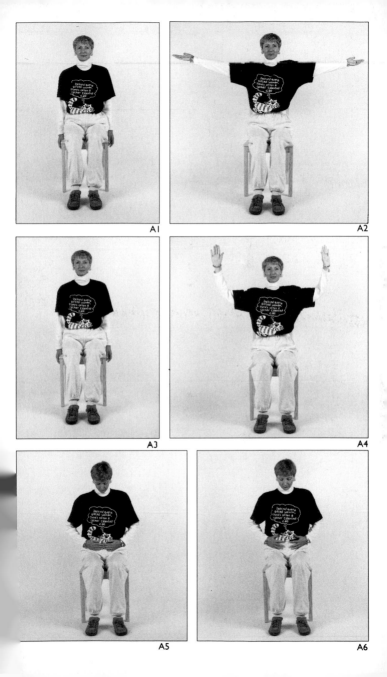

A1

A2

A3

A4

A5

A6

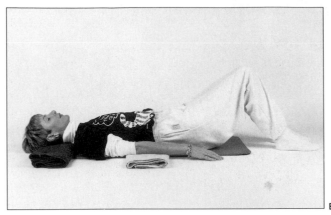

B1

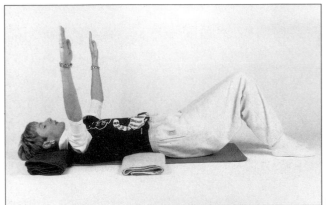

B2

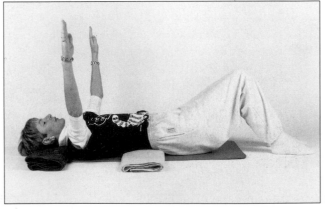

B3

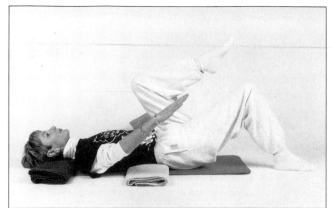

B4

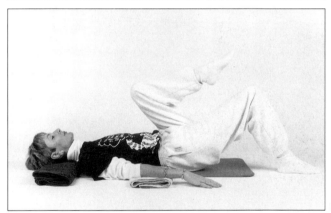

B5

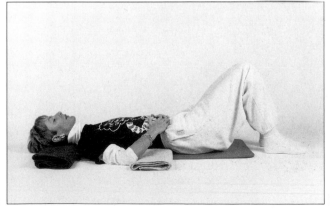

B6

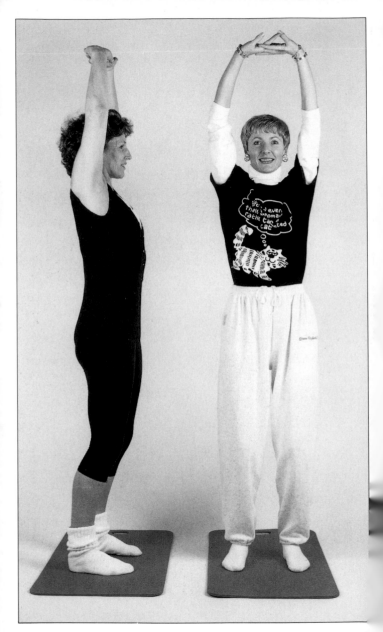

C

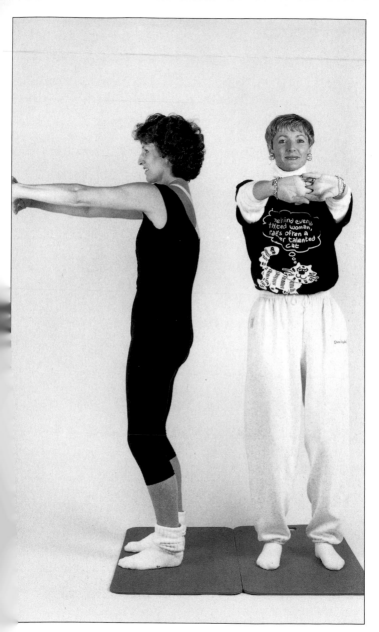

D

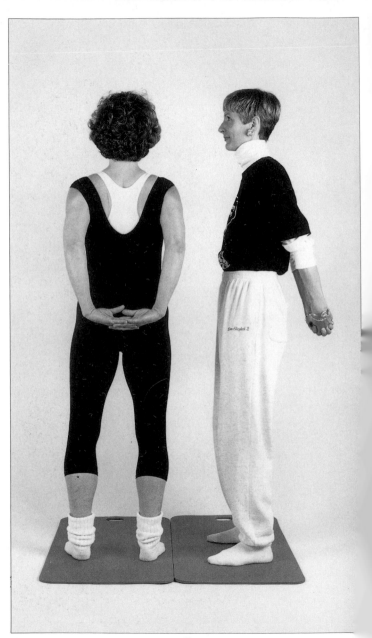

E

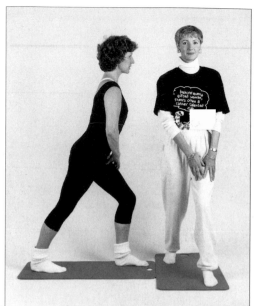

F

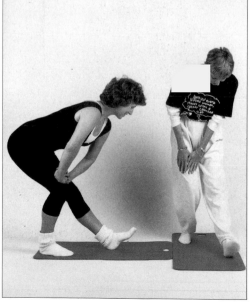

G

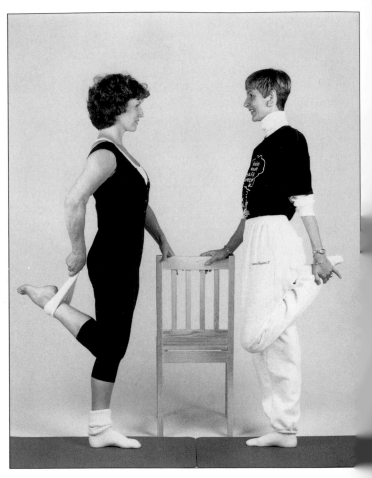

H

world. A neglected pillow may be 10 per cent heavier than its weight when new because of the accumulated house-dust mites, dead skin and allergen-loaded dung! Where did you say you were sleeping tonight?

*** Allergy sufferers will find more information in the Products and Services section on page 346 and in Further Reading on page 339.

*** Look after your teeth with a non-fluoride toothpaste but avoid tooth *powders*. Their abrasive character can wear down and release the mercury amalgam which is now known to be toxic. The health food store has plenty of suitable alternatives.

*** If your dentist recommends a filling, ask about alternatives to mercury amalgam. There is now a huge amount of unignorable evidence to show that cramming our teeth with the second most toxic substance next to plutonium is not a health bonus. If you are fobbed off, find another dentist. However, having existing mercury fillings replaced should only be considered with the assistance of a dentist who has plenty of experience in the art. If not done properly and carefully, drilling them out may cause more problems than leaving well alone.

*** Don't allow yourself to be subjected to unnecessary X-ray investigation. These routine tests are generally over-prescribed and are often carried out using out-of-date equipment which is poorly maintained. If your doctor deems a dose is absolutely necessary, make sure that you increase your intake of Vitamin C (one gram three times daily) for two days before and for seven days after any exposure. If possible, ask that your reproductive organs are protected from X-rays during examination.

*** Check your period protection. As a health practitioner, and in view of the seriousness of Toxic Shock Syndrome, I would always prefer to avoid tampons totally. It is also important to steer clear of any press-on towels or panty shields which do not specifically state that they are free of plastic and made without chlorine bleach. Pester your chemist, drug store and supermarket to stock environmentally-friendly products. More info. under Environment on page 347.

*** In addition to a healthy diet, take a daily multivitamin/mineral complex plus a gram of vitamin C for extra pollution protection. Occasional courses of silymarin – the liver cleansing herb – could also be most beneficial (used in conjunction with practitioner advice, please).

SOURCES OF REFERENCE:

~ Rogers S A. A Practical Approach to the Person with Suspected Indoor Air Quality Problems. *International Clinical Nutrition Review* 1991;11(3):126–30.

~ Abramson M. & Voight T. Ambient Air Pollution and

Respiratory Diseases. *The Medical Journal of Australia* 1991;154:543–53.

~ Gerehard/Ingrid et al. Prolonged Exposure to Wood Preservatives Induces Endocrine and Immunologic Disorders in Women. *American Journal of Obstetrics and Gynaecology* 1991;165(2):487–8.

~ Article by anonymous author published in *Business Week*, 6 April 1992, page 36: Breast cancer and PCBs; a possible link. Also reported by Gaby A. Gaby's Literature Review & Commentary, Pollution and Breast Cancer. *Townsend Letter for Doctors*, Aug/Sep 1992, page 691.

~ Health Education Authority leaflet: Breathing Other People's Smoke; The Effects of Passive Smoking. Undated.

~ Papers and notes taken from conference on The Toxic Chemical Load, Sydney, Australia, 23–24 July 1993.

~ Smith Bob L. Nutrients in Modern Agriculture. *Journal of Applied Nutrition* 1993;45:35–39. Also reported in *Townsend Letter for Doctors* November 1993, page 1047.

~ Notes provided by Indoor Air International Association following conference on Volatile Organic Compounds, London, England, 27–28 October 1993.

~ Bawdon F. X-rays – diagnostic excess. *What Doctors Don't Tell You* 1993;4(6):1–3.

~ *The Food Magazine*, Feb/Apr 1992, page 4.

~ *The Food Magazine*, Feb/Apr 1993, page 7.

~ The Annual Report of the Working Party on Pesticide Residues 1991. Published by HMSO 1992.

~ Best S. Power lines – the leukaemia link. *What Doctors Don't Tell You* 1994;5(3):1–3.

~ Randolph Theron G. Fatigue and Weakness of Allergic Origin (Allergic Toxemia) to be differentiated from

'Nervous Fatigue' or Neurasthenia. *Annals of Allergy* 1945;3:418–30.

~ Rowe A H. Allergic Fatigue and Toxemia. *Annals of Allergy* 1959;17:9–18.

~ Rowe A H. Allergic Toxemia and Fatigue. *Annals of Allergy*. 1950;8:72–9.

Weinberg E G. Allergic Tension Fatigue Syndrome. *Annals of Allergy*. 1973;31:209–11.

7

Feeling TATT? (Tired all the Time?)
Should You Tell the Doctor?

'Doctors are mostly imposters. The older a doctor is the more
venerated he is, the more he must pretend to know everything.
Of course, they grow worse with time. Always look for a doctor
who is hated by the best doctors. Always seek out a bright
young doctor before he comes down with nonsense.

Thornton Wilder (1897–1975)
US novelist and dramatist

Episodes of the tiredness syndrome come around almost
more frequently than tv repeats of *Easter Parade* or *White
Christmas*. But are they serious enough to bother the
doctor?

The answer could be a lemon. If unexplained exhaustion has plagued you for several weeks or your current
level of health – or rather, not-so health – has reached the
stage when it is worrying you, then you could be labelled
a lemon if you don't check it out with your general practitioner. It doesn't necessarily follow that you will need
medical treatment but a few basic tests and a full examination can do wonders to put your mind at rest.

There is certainly a place in health care for the maxim
'If it ain't broke, don't fix it.' That doesn't mean there is
no place for professional medical advice. Discovering that
there is nothing seriously wrong is surely a diagnosis
worth celebrating! Lift a heavy weight off the mind and
who knows how many problems might disappear?

It's a comforting fact that the majority of conditions are either self-limiting (they get better anyway) or will respond to the simplest of dietary and lifestyle changes. One doctor I spoke with suggested that many a symptom would be despatched swiftly by a day off, a warm bath, an early night, a deep breath and a glass of water – although he didn't say in which order! For most kinds of cave-in, the best treatments are undemanding and effective. Rest, good food, fresh air, friends (real ones), relaxation, Vitamin C, homoeopathic first aid, no housework, a holiday, having the kids adopted (only joking!), deciding on a soft spot for the mother-in-law . . . A swamp, perhaps (still joking?).

For a few conditions, however, medical support, diagnosis and intervention may by required. Fatigue can be a common denominator (possibly even the only *initial* symptom) in any number of illnesses. Overactive or underactive thyroid, multiple sclerosis, high blood pressure (hypertension), iron deficiency, diabetes and heart disease are a few of the more serious reasons for feeling TATT.

Whilst the messages we get from our bodily systems can be a useful 'gut instinct' guide to what ails us, self-diagnosis is not always to be recommended.

So, don't be nervous about bothering the doctor if any of the following apply to you. The symptoms are not definitive and are included as indicators only. And, hypochondriacs please note: it doesn't mean that anything *not* included isn't important or that all symptoms in the list indicate serious illness!

???	Severe tiredness of more than three months' duration which hasn't responded to rest
???	Sudden weight-loss (without dieting)
???	Unexplained weight-gain of more than ten pounds in the last three months
???	Fluctuating body temperature
???	Recent/abnormal sensitivity to heat or cold
???	Unusually pale skin or pale nails
???	Vertigo or dizziness
???	Persistent nausea
???	Unexplained/persistent vomiting
???	Recurring indigestion
???	Rapid heartbeat
???	Any change in bowel habit
???	Blood in urine or stools
???	Painful urination
???	Frequent night-time visits to the bathroom
???	Any kind of lump, bump or swelling
???	Moles which have changed shape or bleed
???	Aching or pain, particularly in the chest or arms
???	Constant, unquenchable thirst
???	Loss of appetite – or excessive hunger
???	Night sweats
???	Bleeding from anywhere – except normal menstruation
???	Shortness of breath, especially after climbing stairs

LOW BLOOD PRESSURE (bp) deserves special and separate mention here since its effects can be extremely fatiguing. In the United Kingdom, United States and Canada, a low bp is generally regarded as acceptable – even beneficial – whilst on the European continent, doctors are more likely to view low blood pressure (called hypotension) as a treatable 'problem'. It's an interesting thought that whether you are sick or not could be entirely dependent upon where your doctor went to med school!

Conventional wisdom has it that it's better to have bp readings in the low-to-normal range; also that a lower measurement probably means a longer life (except in some cases of heart disease where blood flow is affected).

More critical cases of low blood pressure can be part and parcel of a number of serious illnesses but, in its *mild* form, is not believed to be life-threatening. In spite of this asset, it can be annoying if the symptoms prevent sufferers from functioning efficiently, especially first thing in the morning when readings can be particularly low. Even simple tasks such as vacuuming, picking anything up from the floor, lifting a small child or getting up from a chair or out of the bath tub too quickly, can bring on unpleasant feelings of nausea, dizziness, fainting, weariness, lethargy, exhaustion, whooshing noises in the ears and headache. One sufferer compared low blood pressure symptoms to rushing headfirst and upside down through a dark, windy tunnel.

Self-help tips include regular relaxation, deep breathing and stretching exercises, increasing water intake, eating regularly and taking care not to miss meals. Vitamin, mineral and herbal supplements which give support to the adrenal system, such as low dose B complex, chromium, ginseng and liquorice, are sometimes recommended. (Similar supplement complexes have also been shown to be helpful in the treatment of thyroid imbalance.) However, I would emphasize, yet again, the potential dangers of taking larger than necessary doses and the false economy of using poor quality products. More information about nutrient supplements can be found on pages 307 and 355.

IRON-DEFICIENCY ANAEMIA is said to be one of the most common nutrient deficiencies and, like low blood pressure, is routinely associated with – you've guessed it again – lack of energy. Women who suffer with heavy periods may also put up with severe tiredness and lethargy, not realizing that their blood loss is causing iron deficiency. So tell your GP, especially if you are experiencing shortness of breath. However, unless a blood test has shown that you are low in iron and your GP recommends that you take extra iron as a supplement – DON'T. Iron overload can be very dangerous indeed. Furthermore, many of the iron pills available are, generally, poorly absorbed and can be irritating to the gut and constipating in the extreme! Unfortunately, the most commonly prescribed iron – ferrous sulphate – falls into this category. One of the reasons it blackens your stools is because most of it ends up in your bowel (to be passed out as waste) rather than in your blood where it is needed.

Don't panic. There are alternatives. For starters, it's good if your diet contains a variety of iron-rich foods from natural sources but better to avoid foods which are 'fortified' with added iron. So check pack labels. Steer clear of iron tonics and other iron supplements unless your doctor has tested the iron levels in your blood and advised that extra iron is absolutely necessary. You'll find a list of foods rich in iron on pages 319–320.

Important notes:

1. If you are involved in active sports or regular workouts, bear in mind that you will probably be using *more* iron and may need to be a little more vigilant about intake. If, despite a good diet which includes a regular variety of the items on pages 319–320, you are suffering with persistent tiredness, breathing problems, heavy periods or if menstruation just isn't happening, then see your GP for a check-up and blood test.

2. The oft printed phrase *'Keep all supplements and medications away from children'* means what it says. Even a low dose iron tablet could kill a small child. Prescription iron tablets are sometimes sugar coated and look like sweets!

3. I came across one report which expressed concern at the number of 'fortified' foods (those which have iron added by the manufacturer) that are now available, since *excessive* iron from supplemented sources may retard growth and increase the risk of heart disease, diabetes and cancer. Children's diets sometimes contain a significant proportion of such foods but may not include so many from completely natural sources. Since iron deficiency is believed to be so widespread, it could be said that iron from anywhere is better than taking too little. A varied diet which includes a goodly proportion of foods naturally rich in iron seems to be the answer.

THYROID PROBLEMS: the thyroid gland acts as a thermostat to control body temperature and has been compared to a power generator which energizes the system. When it misbehaves, a thyroid gland may become 'hyper' and overreactive – or sluggish and underfunctioning; both situations are common. But, in my experience, the very word 'thyroid' clicks in most people's minds with weight increase, a slowed metabolism or lack of energy – in other words, underactivity.

Here is the difference between the two conditions:

An **underactive thyroid** is one which is not producing enough of the hormones *thyroxine* and *tri-iodothyronine*. There may also be a lack of iodine, the nutrient needed to produce thyroid hormones. Known as *hypothyroidism* (or *myxoedema*), this kind of malfunction can result in lethargy, depression, hair loss, loss of sex drive, constipation, persistent infections, high cholesterol, high blood pressure, dry skin and weight gain. Sufferers may complain of feeling generally run down and of increased sensitivity to the cold but often find the problems relating to overweight the most difficult to handle. I hope that the information here – together with that provided in the chapter on Eating for Energy – will prove to be helpful.

An **overactive thyroid** (called *hyperthyroidism* or *thyrotoxicosis*) means an overproduction of those same hormones. Weight loss (despite normal eating), rapid heart beat, racing or irregular pulse, looser bowel movements, breathlessness, sweating, muscle weakness and a dislike of hot weather are common symptoms.

THE CAUSES?

As with so many health problems, a single cause for thyroid imbalance has yet to be isolated. Heredity, poor digestion, poor absorption or inadequate supply of certain vitamins and minerals, too little *quality* protein in the diet, smoking, stress, pituitary gland dysfunction, yo-yo dieting, fluoride excess, certain medications – all these things have been linked to thyroid breakdown. Dr Christine Page suggests that underactivity of the thyroid may be coupled to the need for change, together with a certain resistance and frustration. I have found that some sufferers admit to feeling 'trapped' and unable to have a break from family and other obligations in order to give themselves a little personal priority. Those with overactive thyroid are often involved in many different tasks at one time and may use their 'busy-ness' as an excuse to avoid addressing their own personal creative needs. Activities such as art classes, pottery, languages, literature, poetry and music can provide therapeutic outlets. The chapter Power Up Against Stress also contains quite a few tips which may be helpful for anyone with a thyroid problem. Self-care is especially important.

MEDICAL TREATMENT

If your GP suspects a thyroid problem s/he may suggest sending some blood away for analysis. Unfortunately – and this is generally accepted – the yardstick used for thyroid testing is not always as exact or precise as it might be, especially if your results fall within the lower limits of 'normal'. In other words, a reading at the extreme end of low could still be read as 'normal', leaving a mild thyroid malfunction undetected and untreated.

In the case of an *under*active thyroid gland, the preferred medical prescription will be for thyroid hormone. Where the gland is *over*active, drugs which *suppress* thyroid hormone are usually given. In either case, dosage is likely to be dependent upon the blood test results and should, at all times, be carefully monitored; frequent check-ups and follow-up tests are absolutely essential so that individual patient requirements can be administered and adjusted accordingly. It's all too easy to get sucked into a 'repeat prescription' routine with only occasional consultations.

DR BRODA BARNES

A pioneer in the treatment of hypothyroidism in the United States is Dr Broda Barnes who overcame the quirks of existing methods by introducing his Basal Temperature Test, a simple procedure which patients could carry out at home with an ordinary mercury thermometer. If temperamental temperature control is a feature in thyroid malfunction, he reasoned, then body temperature ought to be able to indicate the level of metabolic function. When temperatures are persistently lower than average – and accompanied by any of the hypothyroid symptoms described above – then Dr Barnes would consider that the thyroid was underfunctioning and treat accordingly.

Whilst his test is listed in the American Physician's

Desk Reference, the majority of doctors – especially those in the UK and Europe – are completely unaware of his research. As his work shows, drug medication is not always required. Borderline thyroid problems do, in many cases, respond to simple dietary intervention. Treatment may also require the use of certain vitamins and minerals – with, or without, small amounts of natural thyroid hormone (not to be confused with glandular extracts).

OVERWEIGHT THYROID?

Where there is stubborn excess weight gain, standardized extract of the Garcinia Cambogia fruit, taken in supplement form, has proven to be helpful. *Garcinia Cambogia* is available without prescription but should be used in conjunction with professional dietary advice. Details on page 330.

LOOK AFTER YOUR LIVER

Doing whatever you can to keep the liver healthy is always important but, according to the laws of naturopathy, could be even more so if you suffer with thyroid problems. The liver is responsible for dealing not only with waste and metabolic toxins but also with hormones. In an overloaded liver, there is always a good chance that 'used' hormones won't be broken down and/or properly recycled, which could, in turn, affect those produced by the thyroid gland. In addition, a 'junked-up' liver can inhibit the production of detoxifying enzymes. There is also the suggestion that processed polyunsaturated spreads and oils may not be helpful as they could interfere with the production, transport and conversion of thyroid hormones.

Whilst orthodox experts do not, as a rule, go along with this theory, they are likely to agree that the liver plays a major role in detoxification. Naturopaths report improvements in thyroid patients when liver function is also taken into account.

Increasing fresh fruits and vegetables, drinking plenty of water, cutting out as many chemicals and additives from the diet as possible, going easy on the alcohol and the caffeine, avoiding cow's milk and hydrogenated vegetable oils and adding live yoghurt and extra virgin oil are all helpful moves. In addition, those already on thyroid medication may still benefit from low dose vitamin, mineral and/or herbal combination supplements.

A couple of days each month on fresh fruits, vegetables, salads and water – avoiding all concentrated proteins and starches – can also give the liver and the rest of the digestive system a well-earned rest. The chapter, Tired or Toxic? has more information.

WHAT TO DO

If you suspect that your thyroid is misbehaving, first see your doctor. If results are indeterminate and symptoms persist, ask for the test to be repeated. If you are still no farther forward, you could benefit from consulting a practitioner who is familiar with Dr Barnes's studies, the Basal Temperature Test and associated suitable nutritional treatment. See How to Find a Practitioner on page 352 and Further Reading on page 344 for more information.

HYPOGLYCAEMIA
If sudden hunger, poor co-ordination, coldness and collapse of energy happen to you more often that you'd like – and other possible health disorders have been been eliminated – it's worth considering the likelihood that you could be suffering from *hypoglycaemia*. This 'energy assassin' is also sometimes referred to as *low blood sugar disease*.

CONTENTIOUS DEBATE

Hypoglycaemia falls into two basic categories, termed Organic or Reactive. *Organic hypoglycaemia*, where blood glucose levels are persistently low, occurs relatively infrequently – for example, in alcoholism, chronic liver disease, disorders of the endocrine system or heavy metal poisoning. In all these conditions, hypoglycaemic indications could be expected to be fairly obvious and low blood sugar easy to spot.

However, an increasing number of studies suggest that *reactive hypoglycaemia* (also sometimes called *functional hypoglycaemia*) may affect far greater numbers of the population. They may not be troubled by the illnesses listed above but are, nevertheless, incapacitated by a set of extremely debilitating and exhausting symptoms.

SO WHAT IS HYPOGLYCAEMIA?

The reactive 'hypo' is described in medical dictionary

terms as an abnormal condition in which the person's blood glucose level rises after eating (as it should do) but then falls below normal. As a direct result of there being too little circulating glucose (don't forget it is the body's main fuel supply), brain function may be affected, reaction time slowed and performance impaired.

However, there is much disagreement on the prevalence of this type of *hypoglycaemia*. The popular view is that the condition has reached epidemic proportions. One report (from the American Department of Health, Education and Welfare) estimates that as many as one in every two people may be suffering from this kind of low blood sugar disease. Another suggests that *hypoglycaemia* is 'very rare and that many people experience low blood sugar levels without symptoms'. It has also been reported that *hypoglycaemia* is a 'spurious explanation for psychologically caused problems'.

A paper published in the *Journal of Behavioural Medicine* referees that the truth may fall somewhere in between. The difficulty for some doctors is that, whilst they accept the existence of *organic hypoglycaemia*, there is a tendency to see *reactive hypoglycaemia* as 'not a significant problem' – or even a problem at all.

There is also no medical agreement on the principles for properly diagnosing *reactive hypoglycaemia* so that symptoms might easily be misdiagnosed, dismissed or ignored.

One of the difficulties may be that, in tests for *reactive hypoglycaemia*, the fasting glucose (the level measured in your blood after they have denied you your food for a nightmarish twelve hours!) *may not show up as abnormal*. In other words, you complain of low blood sugar, the doctor does a test, the results are normal so the opinion is that they can't find anything wrong with you. You're nuts. Don't you just love it.

> At last a light at the end of the tunnel in your feature on hypoglycaemia. I have been a sufferer since my school days and have had to live with many ignorant comments from doctors and specialists telling me it is 'all in the mind'. However, I have now actually been diagnosed with reactive hypoglycaemia. I am 41 years old.
>
> *Letter from reader*

A scan of the literature reveals many disagreements and contradictions. However, the overall consensus is that *reactive hypoglycaemia* does exist and does produce a range of disagreeable symptoms. In addition, there is a belief that hypoglycaemic symptoms are not only triggered when glucose levels fall to their lowest point but by the frequency and rate of fall. In other words, it isn't how low it goes but how often it goes low – if you see what I mean.

In hypoglycaemia, symptoms usually occur when the body has been without food for anything from ninety minutes to four or five hours. How many of them relate to YOU?

Sudden and dramatic loss of energy (and how!)
The 'shakes'
Feeling spaced out
Feeling lightheaded or dizzy
Poor short-term memory (what memory?)

Palpitations

Cravings (chocolate bingeing ring any bells?)

Attacks of yawning

Cobwebbed consciousness – feeling as though you are fighting through some kind of fog to stay upright

Blurred vision or difficulty focusing

Drowsiness – particularly between meals

Hunger headaches

Anxiety and panic attacks (terrifying)

Feeling 'the blues'

Confused thinking (Hmmmmmmmm?)

Dropping or bumping into things (hypos can be expensive as well as bruising!)

Gnawing hollowness in the stomach

Yuck!

Sudden shivering

Can't get warm

Extreme coldness of hands and feet

Excessive perspiration

Night sweats

Need for frequent meals during the day

Waking up ravenously hungry during the night

Excessive thirst

Over-breathing (hyperventilation)

Unexplained irritability

In more serious cases, nightmares, verbal abuse, physical violence and blackouts may overcome normally placid and well-behaved individuals who, without realising the dangers of possible coma, have allowed their blood glucose to fall almost beyond reach. In such circumstances, sufferers are unlikely to be consciously aware of their behaviour.

The key words in the above list are 'yuck' – which is how you feel when a hypo hits you – and 'dramatic loss of energy', which is what you end up with. You're moving along OK thanks and, suddenly, you can't go any farther. You've been staring at the task in hand for at least ten minutes and your brain won't work. You feel like grim death. You have to stop, rest, eat, something, anything. Your blood glucose levels are through the floor; your body has run out of fuel. Not surprisingly, you're exhausted. You seek professional help but no-one takes you seriously. Seems familiar?

From this list of symptoms, it is also clear to see how easy it can be to wrongly diagnose hypoglycaemia as anxiety neuroses. If you present to your doctor or casualty department with such symptoms as fast heartbeat, rapid breathing, profuse sweating, trembling and feeling afraid, once they have eliminated other more obvious possibilities, the chances are that diagnosis could come down to 'panic attack', 'ataxia' or, worse still, 'can't find what's wrong so it must be . . .' (dear, oh, dear, here we go again) '. . . all in the mind'. Great heavens, the phrase itself is enough to make you crazy!

A DIABETIC FACT OF LIFE

Mention the word 'hypo' to almost any diabetic and they will know at once what you mean. Experienced in their own treatment, most are well practised in how to prevent or to handle the hypo swiftly and safely. But as the letter – written in 1993 and typical of so many sufferers – confirms, see-sawing blood sugar levels affect non-diabetics too, a discovery first recorded over seventy years ago following research by Dr Seale Harris in Birmingham, Alabama, USA.

STOKING THE SYSTEM

Glucose is the premier fuel which provides energy to the muscles and fodder to the brain cells and nervous system; in other words, the bits that make you move and think. This fuel is extracted from the food we eat and, either put to immediate use or tucked away in the tissues until it is needed. Levels are kept on an even keel by the endocrine (hormonal) system; you know – the one that gets blamed for everything that ails you, especially if you're female! Organs of main involvement are the liver, the pancreas and the adrenal glands.

When you feel peckish, that sensation is the result of a message from the hunger centre in your brain telling you that your blood glucose levels have fallen a touch and need replenishing. But in hypoglycaemia, the hormones which raise and lower blood glucose are seriously overworked with the result that the balancing system breaks down. Indeed, another name for hypoglycaemia is *hyperinsulinism*

— overproduction of the hormone insulin, whose main function is to lower the levels of blood glucose. Too much insulin doesn't only mean that blood glucose falls too far. Clinical research points to a connection between over-production of insulin, high blood pressure and heart disease. If the pancreas is allowed to become 'trigger happy', the long-term consequences of untreated hypoglycaemosis might also be a precursor to diabetes.

HYPOGLYCAEMIA – SOME POSSIBLE CAUSES

1. Persistently inadequate intake of calories – i.e. as in low calorie weight loss diets:

Dieters are a number one definite at-risk group from hypoglycaemia. Since a hypo attack is often tantamount to an energy crisis, it perhaps explains why dieters also suffer so much from chronic tiredness. Cut calories too far for too long and you can't possibly be feeding the body enough fuel to keep blood glucose levels stable.

2. And then there are the c-r-a-v-i-n-g-s!!!!

The cravings associated with dieting and with hypoglycaemia (most often for sweetness but sometimes also for salty food) happen because the body knows that very low blood glucose is, in the worst case scenario, a danger to life. You didn't get enough to eat on that stupid diet, remember? The 'safety net' is your own internal messenger service which calls up instant sugar supplies. In emergencies such as this, it is the quickest way to raise the levels of glucose in the blood. You respond by grabbing the chocolate, sugar is absorbed pronto and immediate danger is averted.

Picture what happens if you keep this up.

Too little food = too little fuel

Levels of glucose are used up more quickly

You don't have enough fuel to keep going

You feel terrible

Your stamina slumps

Your brain and nervous system go on holiday

Out comes the chocolate

Blood glucose rises rapidly

You feel fine for a few minutes

Insulin shoots out from the pancreas

Blood glucose crashes

Your adrenal glands have exhausted themselves trying
    to restore the status quo

You don't have enough fuel to keep going

You feel terrible

Your stamina slumps . . .

De da de dum dumb. The emphasis here is on 'dumb'.

Persistent 'on/off' low calorie dieting is a dumb thing to do; a mug's game – unless you want to shove your metabolic rate into bottom gear, ride your blood sugar on a roller coaster and put your health at very serious risk. Don't do it. Please don't do it. If you'd welcome more information on how to stop, follow the dietary advice on pages 173–176.

3.   Missing breakfast and skipping lunch; both common activities in the stressed – or the overweight, straining to lose a few extra pounds:

It is common for those who are overworked to miss out

on meals. But the gain is short-term. Lack of food means less energy *and* reduced performance. And don't imagine for a moment that foregoing a meal or two – or more – will help you to maintain weight loss. Short-term gain again. You might shed a pound or two but it won't be for long.

4.   A fondness for sugar:

Pandering to a sweet tooth and ignoring a dependence on sugary foods is a daredevil way to increase the risk of adrenal exhaustion, hypoglycaemia and/or diabetes – and of your teeth falling out! Almost every organ in the body will be working overtime. Like machinery which is never allowed to rest, breakdown becomes more likely. Adult hypoglycaemia may also be programmed early on in life. Bribe the baby with too many sweet treats and the corruption of adult health could be the consequence. Hyperactivity in children – and in adults – has been linked more than once to the 'pure, white and deadly'. The junk food diets so popular in teenage years are also likely to lay the groundwork for later health problems.

5.   Addiction to stimulants such as coffee, tea, cola, salt, sugar or alcohol:

In reasonable, sensible quantities, none of the above is likely to cause severe health problems – but in excess they will put enormous strain on the system as well as using up vitamins and minerals – increasing the likelihood of outright deficiency. Too much tea, for example, can rob the body of its iron stores which, in turn, can lead to iron-deficiency anaemia – the main symptom of which is persistent tiredness. Alcohol in excess is a nutrient-robber and can disturb many aspects of liver function – one of the organs which figures so prominently in balancing your blood glucose! Other stimulants may, directly or indirectly, overload the pancreas and adrenal system, increasing the risk of hypoglycaemia and exhaustion.

6.   Deficiency of B vitamins:

The B group vitamins are essential for glucose production and for the release of energy but are often destroyed by cooking and food processing. Wholefoods contain far richer sources of B vitamins than their poor factory-refined relatives. Check labels and steer clear of anything which is 'fortified' or 'enriched' as this generally indicates a processed food!

7.   Deficiency of trace minerals:

Chromium, lost when food is refined, has been confirmed by a number of well documented studies to be below normal levels in large numbers of the population. Without chromium, insulin just can't do its job properly. Research reinforces the experience of many practitioners who find that low dose supplementation of the right kind of chromium can be enormously beneficial in the treatment of hypoglycaemia and cravings. Page 321 has more information.

Zinc, another trace element often lacking in the average diet, is also needed for effective insulin production. But don't be tempted to supplement any nutrient either in large amounts or in isolation. Check out the chapter on Increasing the Nutrients in Your Diet.

8.   Deficiency of magnesium:

This mineral is also at risk from damage by the food refining process and yet is essential for blood glucose control. But bear in mind the comments about supplementation of poor quality magnesium supplements mentioned in the section on ME.

9.   Excessive mental overload, physical stress or trauma:

Stress puts additional strain on the endocrine system, particularly the adrenal glands which also produce glucose-balancing hormones and so may predispose a stressed person to hypoglycaemic symptoms. Add stress to low blood glucose and you have an instant recipe for being completely shattered.

10.   Long-term use of certain medications, i.e. diuretic drugs, tranquillizers, the contraceptive pill or HRT:

If you think that your medicine is upsetting your blood glucose, ask your GP or hospital clinic for advice. If you're not satisfied, don't be afraid to push for a second opinion.

11.   Familial or hereditary hypo:

The condition can also run in families and may be more likely where there is a history of diabetes, obesity, alcoholism or prolonged stress.

12.   Poor digestion:

Poor digestion can lead to inadequate absorption of the very nutrients needed to produce energy and keep blood glucose in balance. Improving the efficiency of the digestive system can be a vital factor in a great many conditions, including hypoglycaemia and thyroid disorders. More information can be found from page 267.

13.   Reliance on artificial sweeteners:

Given the advertising hype, it is understandable that people might turn to artificial sweeteners in the belief that these are healthier than sugar. But watch out! Investigations suggest that not only do sweeteners disturb the appetite as much as sugar but also that, despite assurances, these chemicals may produce unacceptable side effects and harbour as yet undiscovered health risks. The jury is still out but, until they return with a majority verdict, perhaps caution is the best option?

HELP FOR THE HYPO

*** The good news is that *reactive hypoglycaemia* is not difficult to treat nutritionally. Indeed, some experts are convinced that it survives and thrives only because of our dependence upon high sugar diets. One study suggests that 'clinicians can assist their hypoglycaemic patients in developing individually tailored self-management programs [and that] people experiencing symptoms can learn which foods cause symptoms to arise and the time interval between eating and onset.' Certainly, there are plenty of easy-to-follow self-help things you can do which should effect a real improvement in the way you've been feeling lately. From 'yuck' to 'yippee', I guess. I hope the following hints are helpful.

***   If you suspect hypoglycaemia, the first step is to ask your GP for a health check. If nothing else, it's important to eliminate the possibility of any other conditions which have similar symptomatology.

A single blood glucose test carried out at the surgery or health clinic may not be sufficient or accurate enough to give useful guidance on whether or not hypoglycaemia is a problem for you. You may therefore be referred to hospital for something called a GTT (Glucose Tolerance Test) which monitors an individual's glucose levels over a period of several hours. However, even these findings may not be conclusive since they measure only the glucose levels and not the insulin. Like intermittent faults in a piece of household equipment which *never* show up when the engineer calls to investigate, low blood glucose has an irritating habit of testing normal when anyone in a white coat appears with a hypodermic.

Some doctors now believe that a G/ITT (Glucose/Insulin Tolerance Test) gives more accurate and reliable measurements.

***   All hypoglycaemics must get into the breakfast habit. If you think breakfast is a turn-off, then eat *something* – even if it is only a piece of fruit – as soon as you can face food – and then keep up your intake of fruit throughout the morning if that is all you can manage. Don't, don't, don't go all the way to your lunch break on an empty stomach. That's an order! Nag, nag, nag!

***   Carry snacks with you if there is a chance you might have to miss a meal.

***   If you are hungry, eat something. Don't be regulated by someone else's meal times.

***   Don't miss meals. Enjoy snacks mid-morning

and mid-afternoon. Ignore the mind-set which taught you that eating meant putting on weight. Eating little and often is better for weight balance.

*** Eat a light snack about an hour before bedtime. This is good insurance against waking hungry during the night.

*** Avoid added sugar totally and completely; cut right down on any foods which contain sugar or white flour, such as sweet biscuits, cakes, pastries or chocolate – and artificial sweeteners which, remember, can disturb the appetite just as dramatically as sugar.

*** Cut down on coffee, tea, cola and salt but do it gradually. Becoming a goody two shoes overnight could trigger serious withdrawal symptoms!

*** Although some of us are now relying heavily on the advice that red wine might be good for the heart and that the natural silicon found in beer may be able to reduce the aluminium in our systems, it's worth remembering that alcohol can make hypoglycaemic symptoms worse. If you drink, avoid excesses, steer clear of the hard stuff, try not to drink on a completely empty stomach and take wine only with meals.

*** Rule out the possibility of food intolerances. A number of practitioners have observed that sensitivity to certain foods aggravates – and may even be the cause of – hypoglycaemia in some people. The section on pages 284–285 contains a general guide to the foods which are the most troublesome.

*** Try food combining. To the apparent chagrin of a few dietitians, not mixing proteins and starches at the same meal really does seem to help balance blood glucose levels and 'hit the hypo where it hurts'. Some fitness teachers now recommend food combining to their classes simply because of its talent for preventing the hypo attacks so commonly associated with workouts. More information on pages 273–279.

*** On the subject of protein, are you getting enough? If you're not sure, the chapter on Eating for Energy (page 257) should help. Studies show that blood glucose levels in hypoglycaemics are maintained at a more beneficial level where protein intake is slightly higher.

*** Protect yourself from stress; stress damage can increase hypo attacks. Tried and tested tips can be found on pages 27–54.

*** Don't be a slave to low cal dieting. Do it the healthy way on page 257.

*** Make sure your daily intake of food includes a reasonable amount of dietary fibre – especially from pulses, cereals such as oats, rice and rye (not wheat), nuts, fresh fruit and vegetables. Linseeds are a particularly good source of fibre. Remember that extra fibre needs extra fluid; try introducing three glasses of water a day in addition to your usual beverages.

*** Get into the label reading habit. Be especially wary of foods which contain long lists of chemical sounding names and an over-abundance of E numbers. Keep in mind that anything ending in '. . . ose' (maltose, glucose, sucrose, dextrose, etc.) is sugar in disguise.

*** Avoid antacid indigestion remedies and supplements which are labelled calcium carbonate, bonemeal or dolomite. Researchers have found that these products can disturb levels of the trace mineral chromium – one of the most important elements in the maintenance of blood glucose balance.

DON'T IGNORE PERSISTENT SYMPTOMS

One of the major (and justifiable) complaints by doctors is that patients leave things too long before seeking advice. Sometimes we may be nervous about the outcome of a consultation and make the excuse that we're too busy or that there are people with much more serious complaints than ours who deserve priority.

We all know that doctors can be abrupt, aggressive, touchy, egotistical, holier than thou, sometimes frightening, sometimes deaf and sometimes just plain wrong. I've heard enough 'Doctor wouldn't discuss it', 'Doctor doesn't listen', 'Doctor told me to pull myself together' stories to last me a lifetime. In this book, I've shared one or two of the more amusing and one or two of the more alarming ones with you.

Even calling for an appointment can take courage. Although now rare, there was a time when some visits had to be sanctioned by Attila the Receptionist before you were allowed to tiptoe into the consulting room. So terrifying was one particular ogre who reigned supreme during the hormonal hiatus of my teens, the locals said of her that she either frightened you to death or scared your symptoms away thereby rendering the doctor completely superfluous to requirements. Looking back and wondering how she ever got away with it, I guess no-one was brave enough to complain. Certainly not faint-heart cowardy custard me! Nowadays, of course, things are very different.

The receptionists at my present surgery are 180° away from that kind of attitude and deserve medals for the patience they display towards their patients. Birds of a feather obviously do flock together, since the doctor they work with shows similar empathy and expertise.

There are plenty of excellent GPs who are attentive, sympathetic, straightforward, helpful and good at what they do. And we don't always make life easy for them or their staff. We grouch and moan and demand and complain and pull faces but do we ever smile, ask the doctor how s/he is feeling, communicate, communicate or communicate? Hell, no!

It was the great, good and gorgeous Dr Bernie Siegel who reminded us that M.D. does not stand for Medical Deity. It's worth remembering. A few doctors, more than enough consultants – and the odd professor here and there – do have godlike egos but, conversely, we – as patients – have an unfair tendency to expect miracles.

What a successful surgery visit comes down to is contact, conversation and c-o-m-m-u-n-i-c-a-t-i-o-n. That is something we don't do well. We are subjective rather than objective. We are negative, not positive; passive instead of active. Perhaps we don't have the energy! Or the courage? It's your health and your body so tell your GP how you *f-e-e-l*, if it hurts – where it hurts, how often, how severely, etc. Discuss the issues, ask plenty of questions – especially about any prescription which is offered to you, ask how long you should follow the treatment, if there are any other symptoms to look out for, what side effects, what improvements to expect. Doctors don't have all the answers (an article in an issue of the *British Medical Journal* of 1878 alleged that a joint of meat spoiled because a menstruating woman was standing nearby!) but can give important and useful guidance. Doctors are also the ones likely to be dragged out of bed in the middle of the night to people who could have visited the surgery the previous day or waited until morning!

If the condition doesn't improve, go back. It's useless to whinge on about the doctor if we were at fault for failing to find out as much information as possible at the first recce. I have lost count of the number of times that patients have come to my clinic, given me a full history of their prescribed drugs and then admitted that they didn't know what any of the pills were for, what the diagnosis was or even if there was a diagnosis at all.

If you are not satisfied, seek another opinion. Anyone with a doctor problem would do well to contact *What Doctors Don't Tell You* for copies of their special reports on how to obtain the best surgical and medical treatment. (Address on page 340). Invest also in a copy of Stephen Fulder's book *How To Be A Healthy Patient*, published by Hodder & Stoughton. To stick with the status quo when the status quo is not helping your health is a fast track way to becoming even more stressed and fatigued.

SOURCES OF REFERENCE:

~ Johnston L N. Hemochromatosis [iron overload]. Article in *Townsend Letter for Doctors* June 1994;pp582–4.
~ Idjradinata P et al. Adverse effect of iron supplementation on weight gain of iron-replete young children. *Lancet* 1994;343;1252–4.
~ Peat R. Thyroid Misconceptions. Article in *Townsend Letter for Doctors* November 1993;pp1120–2.
~ Wessely S, Nickson J, Cox B. Symptoms of low blood

pressure; a population study. *British Medical Journal* 1990;301:362–5.

~ Lossos A, Argov Z. Orthostatic hypotension induced by vitamin B12 deficiency. *Journal of the American Geriatric Society* 1991;39:601–3.

~ Harris S. Hyperinsulinism and Dysinsulinism. *Journal of the American Medical Association* 1924;83:729.

~ Harris S. The Diagnosis and Treatment of Hyperinsulinism. *Annals of International Medicine* 1936;1010:54.

~ Banovac K, Zakarija M, McKenzie J M. Experience with routine thyroid function testing: abnormal results in 'normal' populations. *Journal of the Florida Medical Association Inc* 1985;72(10):835–9.

~ Flowers S W. Absorption of simple sugars. *Townsend Letter for Doctors* July 1992;594.

~ Taylor L, Rachman S. The effects of blood sugar level changes on cognitive function, affective state and somatic symptoms. *Journal of Behavioural Medicine* 1988;11(3):279–91.

~ Kerr D, Sherwin R S, Pavalkis F, Fayad P B, Sikorski L et al. Effect of caffeine on the recognition of and responses to hypoglycaemia in humans. *Annals of Internal Medicine* 1993;119:799–804.

~ Gaby A R, Wright J V. Nutritional Regulation of Blood Glucose. *Journal of Advancement in Medicine* 1991;4(1):57–67.

~ Shah S et al. The significance of the flat glucose tolerance test. *Journal of the Kansas Medical Association*; November 1975;263–7.

~ The Slimming Scandal, *The Food Magazine*, Feb/Apr 1992;8–9.

~ Intense Sweeteners Do Not Decrease Appetite. *Obesity 91 Update*. May/June 1991;4.

~ Stebbing J B, Turner M O, Franz K B. Reactive hypoglycaemia and magnesium. *Magnesium Bulletin* 1982;2:131.

~ Wright J V. The Glucose-Insulin Tolerance Test and its relevance to 'essential hypertension' and HDL/LDL cholesterol abnormalities. *International Clinical Nutrition Review* 1990;10(3):381–2.

~ O'Hare J A. The enigma of insulin resistance and hypertension. *American Journal of Medicine* 1988; 84:505–10.

~ Reaves G M. The role of insulin resistance in human disease. *Diabetes* 1985;37:1595–1606.

~ Editorial: Chromium Deficiency – 90 per cent of your patients may be at risk. Report in *The American Chiropractor*, Sept/Oct 1992;22–4.

~ Anderson R A et al. Chromium supplementation of humans with hypoglycaemia. Fed. Proc; 1984;43:471.

~ Hudspeth W J, Peterson L W, Soli D E, Trimble B A. Neurobiology of the hypoglycaemia syndrome. *Journal of Holistic Medicine* 1981;3(10):60.

~ Anderson R W, Lev-Ran A. Hypoglycaemia: The standard and the fiction. *Psychosomatics* 1985;26:38–47.

~ Hadji-Georgopoulos A, Schmidt M L I, Margolis S, Kowarski A A. Elevated hypoglycaemic index and late hyperinsulinism in symptomatic postprandial hypoglycaemia. *Journal of Clinical Endocrinology and Metabolism* 1980;50:371–6.

~ Hofeldt F D. Reactive hypoglycaemia. *Metabolism* 1975;24:1193–1208.

~ Uhde T W, Vittone B J and Post R M. Glucose tolerance testing in panic disorders. *American Journal of Psychiatry* 1984;141:1461–63.

~ Seaborn C, Stoecker B. Effects of antacid or ascorbic acid on tissue accumulation and urinary excretion of chromium. *Nutrition Research* 1990;10:1401–7.

~ Roberts H J. Potential toxicity due to dolomite and bonemeal. *South Med Journal* 1983;76:556.

~ Prinz R J, Roberts W A, Hantman E. Dietary correlates of hyperactive behaviour in children [effect of sucrose]. *Journal of Consulting Clinical Psychiatry* 1980;48:760.

~ *An Alternative to Psychiatry* by Tuula Tuormaa, The Book Guild, 1991.

~ *Hypothyroidism: The Unsuspected Illness* by Broda Barnes and Lawrence Galton, Harper & Row.

~ *Basics of Food Allergy* by J C Breneman, Charles C Thomas, 1978. Clinical observations suggest that food sensitivities may cause functional hypoglycaemia in 75 per cent of patients.

My thanks also to Sally Bunday of the Hyperactive Children's Support Group for the very helpful research material she has provided.

8

ME – The Energy Killer

You've got flu – and a hangover
And you've just run five miles.
How do you feel?
Like someone with ME.
Taken from the 'Action for ME' information literature

No discussion on the problems of energy could ignore ME, the devastating disease so commonly associated with chronic fatigue and the butt of so much scepticism and ridicule. If you have been diagnosed with ME or suspect you may have the condition, I do hope that the information in this chapter will spike your determination and resolve to 'hang in there' and not be discouraged by disbelievers. I hope, also, that at least some of those who remain sceptical will read these words and open their hearts and minds to the plight of ME sufferers.

ME is an illness which has had to battle long and hard for recognition; indeed, the fight still goes on. It should come as no surprise, therefore, that many patients feel abandoned, forsaken and even friendless. They may be seriously ill, a wheelchair or walking frame their only mode of transport, unable to work or even dress themselves but, because they have no plaster cast, no sling or other obvious sign of physical damage, their condition is rarely taken seriously.

I believe ME is a classic example of a common situation where members of the medical fraternity have continually ignored scientific research, patients' observations and case histories. We shouldn't be surprised. Doctors are used to specifics; in their world, a specific set of symptoms should lead to a specific diagnosis which, in turn, leads to a specific treatment. It's tough if you don't belong; a bit like trying to buy clothes if you are slightly taller, shorter, wider or narrower than the norm. Those who don't fit the bill, whether it be diagnosable illnesses or department store dresses, may find themselves out in the cold and compelled to seek alternatives!

A DISEASE BY MANY OTHER NAMES

Chronic Fatigue Syndrome (CFS)
Chronic Fatigue & Immune Dysfunction or
    Dysregulation Syndrome (CFIDS)
Post-Viral Fatigue Syndrome (PVFS)
Icelandic Disease
Akureyri Disease
Yuppie Flu
Raggedy Ann Disease (who?)
Royal Free Disease . . .

All these terms have been used — correctly or incorrectly and kindly or unkindly — to describe Myalgic Encephalomyelitis or ME.

Even if you have been fortunate enough not to have suffered from this very genuine illness, you will almost undoubtedly know — or have heard of — someone who does.

The first recorded case of ME is said to have been in 1756! However, 200 years ago, such reports were rare.

Today, ME is believed to affect more than 150,000 people in the UK alone. Many famous names have been burdened by the disease, the best known probably being the intrepid and talented Clare Francis, author and round-the-world yachtswoman, who, despite her illness has done so much to encourage recognition of the condition.

ME OR CHRONIC FATIGUE? CONFUSION

The reason for so much confusion in naming the condition may be because, when the acronym 'CFS' was first coined, it was to formally define 'disabling fatigue of at least six months' duration', a scenario which is, of course, familiar also to Myalgic Encephalomyelitis. Chronic Fatigue Syndrome, however, is not a single disease but an umbrella term which covers a number of different conditions which have 'chronic fatigue' as a common denominator. Examples include fibromyalgia, neurasthenia, post-viral debility syndrome and feeling TATT, a fitting acronym for Tired-All-The-Time syndrome. At the time of writing, there are moves afoot in the United States to include glandular fever, panic and anxiety disorders and Lyme disease under the CFS heading.

ME is already categorized by the World Health Organization as 'a disease of the nervous system', a *specific condition primarily associated with physical* factors. A listing applauded by Action for ME, the very pro-active and admirable campaign group, who regard ME as a neurological disorder – a physical, not a psychological problem. However, although ME is officially recognized by the

United Kingdom Department of Health as a 'debilitating and distressing condition' with a physical basis, it is still listed in the UK Department of Social Security (DSS) Disability Handbook alongside Chronic Fatigue Syndrome. Action for ME are campaigning to have this categorization changed so that ME appears under its more accurate definition of 'neurological disorder'.

'ALL IN THE MIND'?

An additional complication is that both ME and Chronic Fatigue Syndrome are still labelled by many doctors and journalists as essentially psychiatric in origin. In doing so, they are rejecting not only sound research but a wealth of clinical evidence. Few people realize that ME and CFS are more common than many other conditions for which the medical services make good provision.

Consider fibromyalgia, a condition where muscles become swollen, sore and often too tender to touch and which is known to cause excruciating discomfort; in severe cases, the slightest pressure or movement brings on muscle spasm, stiffness and pain which can be physically incapacitating. It is relatively easy to diagnose and unlikely to be labelled 'all in the mind'. Why then should the tag apply to ME, a similarly distressing condition which also displays some very painful and severely disabling symptoms? Even the names have similarities (myalgia/myalgic).

However . . . I surmise that those doing the labelling are unlikely to have suffered from ME or any form of CFS. It is unfortunate that some specialists feel quite comfortable about inflicting their views on subjects of which they know so little. There is, I guess, also a 'fear of the unknown' spread amongst their scepticism.

I am reminded of the definition of a specialist:

> A specialist is someone who studies for years and years learning more and more about less and less until, in the final analysis, he knows absolutely everything about very little indeed.

Why a particularly humourless university chair should spring to mind at this precise moment, I really can't imagine!

Strong words, you might say. Unreasonable, even? No, I don't believe so. There are almost too many situations where the master of the sweeping statement, the inevitable expert, is de-cobwebbed and pushed in front of a microphone for his or her supposedly specialist viewpoint. The resulting interview often gives far more credence to one isolated, alleged authority than it does to an entire collection of well-documented information provided by those at the sharp end, the sufferers.

BENEFIT OF THE DOUBT?

But even under those circumstances, it isn't difficult to understand the mistrust of the medical profession of a disease (like ME) which has such wide-ranging symptoms and appears to be affecting an ever-increasing number of people. As one medic – obviously a maestro of the mixed metaphor – puts it, 'ME is about as easy to properly diagnose as trying to find a needle in a haystack of red herrings up a blind alley.' Some physicians also see ME as manna from heaven for malingerers who can pounce on a handful of common, but difficult to verify, symptoms and use them to their own advantage!

Research shows that more than 60 per cent of GPs are unwilling or unable to diagnose ME. But differentiating between the sincere and the spurious is not always that simple. One way of helping doctors to understand ME and to diagnose and treat the condition would be to make sure that they all receive regular updates and the very latest research material. Thus far, however – and to the best of my knowledge and research – the Government does not circulate such information to its health professionals!

LACK OF TRAINING?

Another major stumbling block to accurate diagnosis and willing support, according to Dr Charles Shepherd of the ME Association, is that ME is not included in medical school curricula and neither undergraduates nor post-graduates are made aware of symptoms during their training. However, I am advised by the ME Association that this situation is likely to change in the relatively near future. Let's hope so.

ME MYTHS

Before we go any farther, let's oust a few misconceptions.
1.   Having the odd bout of weariness in amongst

general good health does not mean someone is suffering from ME. When ME strikes, you know it.

2.   Whilst there may be the very occasional shirker who chooses to blame their laziness on ME, this is not generally a condition of malingerers.

3.   ME is not, repeat not, not, not 'Yuppie Flu': a grossly misleading media tag, insulting in the extreme and, in my view, no more relevant to 'yuppies' than any other serious disorder.

> The last thing anyone could associate with an ME patient is being 'upwardly mobile' since restricted mobility is a common ME symptom. A short walk to the post box can lead to days of total exhaustion.

PROBLEMS

During the course of my work, I have met many ME fighters. They have some fascinating stories to tell. Disturbingly, though – and almost without exception – the onset of their illness has been met with scepticism and suggestions of 'swinging the lead'. A few have been lucky enough to find understanding and helpful GPs; others have not been so fortunate.

One patient told me her general practitioner had written on her notes that ME stood for 'Malingerer Every time'. Another was advised by her local surgery that if she bothered the doctor with such nonsense again, he would ask that she be removed from his list (her gain, I would say!).

One particularly distressed young woman was referred

immediately to a psychiatrist (a common curse on ME victims). When she was too ill to keep the appointment (because of severe muscle weakness and pain in her arms, she couldn't lift them up high enough to get her clothes on), the psychiatrist took it upon himself to visit the patient at home and give her a dressing down in front of her family for 'wasting doctors' time'. He recommended that anti-depressants, sleeping tablets and laxatives (!) be prescribed. When she asked why he felt she needed laxatives, he told her 'You're full of crap. Otherwise, there's nothing wrong with you. Pull yourself together and get back to work.'

And before all practitioners of psychiatry flood my publisher's office with hate mail, I don't happen to believe that all psychiatrists are a curse. I just think that it is unreasonable to stick the psychiatric label onto a list of irregular or nonconformist symptoms before every effort has been made to investigate all other possibilities.

Another difficulty is that whilst (too many?) doctors still find difficulty in accepting ME as a real illness, a small number seem to have diagnosed 'probably ME' when no other explanation could be found.

A bit like writing 'probably aspirin' on a bottle of unidentifiable pills!

On the positive side of the coin, I know of a few patients who have had unstinting support from their doctors who, in their turn, have been happy for those patients to use nutritional therapy, relaxation, reflexology, herbal medicines and a variety of other treatments to help their condition. Who could doubt that such support can increase the likelihood of recovery?

NO HELP OR TREATMENT

For too long, help for ME sufferers and research into its treatment has been hampered by indifference and prejudice. Many patients are frustrated by not being given the correct diagnosis (or any diagnosis at all for that matter) or by not finding a doctor willing to treat them. If doctors are unsupportive, it follows that family and friends may be likewise. Unfortunately, society is so conditioned into accepting doctor dictum as gospel that it takes strong resolve indeed to go against the medical view.

And think about this.

If ME were a malingerer's excuse or a front for 'yuppie flu', how many sufferers would have the determination to withstand the flak directed at them by a derisive and mocking family? Shirkers would give it up as a lost cause! ME is prone to strike active, busy people who have good motivation and enjoy their work and their life; a fact which makes it all the harder for sufferers to accept the need for rest and relaxation.

The most usual orthodox view is either complete disregard or to offer psychiatric treatment, *despite sound scientific proof that ME has a genuine physical basis*. By its very nature, ME can be stressing and depressing for its victims and for their families. Perhaps that is the reason why it is so often, erroneously, treated as a depressive illness, even though there is important scientific evidence (see **Ongoing research** p. 195) which demonstrates that ME is *not* the same disorder as depression. Wouldn't you get depressed if you couldn't get out of bed, weren't able to look after yourself or your family or couldn't work for weeks on end? In fact, depression occurs no more often in

ME patients than it does with any other chronic physical illness.

ME RUINS LIVES

Disquieting are the statistics that 80 per cent of those afflicted are believed to never recover fully. Sixty per cent are forced to settle for a limited lifestyle and few can work full-time. In addition, ME causes varying degrees of permanent disablement in two out of every ten sufferers.

I'm sure you will be as shocked as I was to learn that the suicide rate amongst ME patients is high. Shocked but not surprised given the long list of devastating symptoms, the disruption to normal lifestyle, the attendant social upheaval and the unforgivable absence of empathy from so many quarters.

SO WHAT EXACTLY IS MYALGIC ENCEPHALOMYELITIS?

A debilitating disease which may have a viral trigger and which is believed to be connected to malfunctions of the endocrine (hormonal) and nervous systems. Work carried out by psychoneuroimmunology (PNI) specialists at the Division of Psychoimmunology, TGH Psychiatry Center in Tampa, Florida, points to a defect in the body's stress circuit. A link has been discovered between overproduction of stress hormones and elevated levels of an immune system chemical called interleukin 1 (which is, itself, triggered by stress), causing the immune system to overwork. There are many additional theories but, at the time of writing, no-one has been able to pinpoint an exact cause. Indeed, that could prove difficult. ME seems, for all the world, a multifactorial, multifaceted problem.

Influenza, glandular fever, vaccinations, excessive stress or trauma, exposure to pollutants and sensitivity to certain chemicals – all can lay the groundwork for ME or exacerbate symptoms in those already affected by the condition. Onset may be obvious and sudden or gradual and difficult to tie down to any specific event, affecting people in a variety of ways and to different degrees of severity.

Symptoms of ME and Chronic Fatigue Syndrome vary from individual to individual and may include:

muscle fatigue
muscle pain
muscle tenderness
muscle weakness
limbs like lead
severe exhaustion after the lightest of exercise
poor concentration
failing memory
tired eyes
discomfort of eye muscles
difficulty focusing
headaches
head like 'cotton wool'
lethargy
debility

> *poor appetite or frequent hunger*
> *indigestion*
> *nausea*
> *shivering*
> *sweating*
> *constipation*
> *diarrhoea*
> *abdominal discomfort*
> *problems with balance*
> *flatulence*
> *bloating*
> *unrefreshing sleep*
> *sleep disturbance*
> *restless limbs*
> *'electric shock pains'*
> *feeling of 'unrealness'*
> *feeling 'spaced out'*
> and – not surprisingly, as a consequence of all that
> – *mood fluctuations.*

ME patients may also suffer from related conditions such as candida albicans, yeast overgrowth, and myocarditis, (inflammation of the muscular walls of the heart). And as if that weren't enough, ME has been known to bring on or aggravate problems associated with balance, with the ear and the facial nerves; for example, tinnitus (persistent noises in the ears), labyrinthitis (inflammation of otitis interna, the inner ear), Ménière's Disease (disturbed balance sometimes also associated with tinnitus and deafness) and facial pain in the form of trigeminal neuralgia or discomfort in the temporomandibular joint. Lots of long words for very unpleasant conditions.

Allergies, food sensitivities, environmental pollutants, intestinal parasites, disturbed gut flora, leaky gut syndrome, irritable bowel syndrome, antibiotics, vaccinations, junk food diets and food poisoning have been linked with ME. One, all or none could be the perpetrator or the perpetuator.

Dr Maurice Mee Lee, writing in the *Blackmores Communicator* journal (August 1991), believes that chronic fatigue may be triggered or exacerbated by, amongst other things, lack of rest, insufficient holidays from work (workaholics please note), too little protein and too much fat. He also cites liver and gallbladder disease, Ross River fever, cysts on the ovaries or kidneys, mastitis (breast tenderness), skin flare-ups, tonsillitis, glandular fever, lymphadenitis (inflammation of the lymph glands) and lymphangitis (inflammation of the lymphatic vessels) as allied conditions. His CFS patients present with sallow complexions and are more likely to have brown or hazel (green/brown) eyes rather than clear green or blue. Interesting observations.

ONGOING RESEARCH

Much research still needs to be done but recent studies attribute ME to an overactive immune system which would be consistent with a continuing viral infection. The viruses most commonly associated with Chronic Fatigue Syndrome are Epstein-Barr virus (EBV),

Cocksackie B, Herpes Simplex, Cytomegalovirus and the measles virus.

If one or more viruses are discovered to be the major troublemakers (and several have been and are being investigated), then supporting the immune system would make sense. It's well known that viruses are everywhere around us. Many people remain completely immune whilst others succumb. Is it too vain a hope that reducing the risk of (or eradicating) ME and CFS is down to simple preventive measures?

NEW TEST PROCEDURES

Studies by scientists at the University of Newcastle, New South Wales, believe they may have isolated and identified a chemical in the urine of Chronic Fatigue sufferers which could assist in the diagnosis and subsequent treatment of this condition. Although more work still has to be done, researchers hope that, ultimately, the new finding will save a great deal of time, money and anxiety for doctors and patients.

SLEEP DISTURBANCE

Another interesting area of research has developed in connection with sleep disturbance in sufferers of ME and CFS. The good news is that experts see these problems as treatable in most cases. If sleep disturbance is a problem for you, it is possible that the right level of magnesium supplements could be the answer and is an option you might like to discuss with your health practitioner. (The tips in chapter 4 on Sleep apply to anyone with a tiredness problem but may be particularly useful to anyone suffering from CFS or ME.)

DETOXIFICATION

Some therapists believe detoxification plays an important role in the treatment of CFS and ME. In my experience, whilst not everyone who has accumulated high levels of toxicity will necessarily be stricken with ME, it seems to be the case that ME sufferers can be affected detrimentally by toxins in the system. Short but regular periods of 'detox' are certainly worthwhile – particularly for the liver, that busy eliminator of toxins. The liver is often under significant pressure and can benefit greatly from the occasional 'spring clean' using liver cleansing herbs. You will find further information on 'detox' in chapter eleven.

A DEPRESSIVE ILLNESS?

Studies at University College London Medical School seem to have put paid, once and for all, to the antagonists' claim that ME is nothing more than depression. Using state-of-the-art technology, scientists compared the blood flow to and from the brain in depressed patients and in those suffering from ME. The blood flow in ME patients was found to be significantly lower than that in either depressed patients or healthy subjects; confirming again that ME is not 'all in the mind' and that there are physical abnormalities — believed to be connected to an overactive immunity.

CRANIO-SACRAL OSTEOPATHY

A number of ME sufferers have reported significant improvements in their condition following treatment from a Cranial Osteopath. The author wonders if this therapy — already known to be helpful for a range of conditions — works for ME by, amongst other things, improving blood flow to the brain?

ABSENT-MINDED

In addition, impaired blood flow could be one of the factors responsible for poor memory, poor concentration and other similar symptoms so distressing in ME. Forgetting names, faces, where you put something down or why you went into a particular room are common to us all and can even be amusing, but when they happen all the time because of illness, such 'waters of Lethe' can be depressing and disturbing. One person's innocent remark of 'I must think of ways of improving my . . . er . . . memory' explains the problems very well.

A FLAT BATTERY?

Other important work carried out at the world famous

'Jimmy's' (St James's University Hospital, Leeds, Yorkshire, England) suggests that the extreme fatigue experienced by people with ME could be caused by a *mitochondrial dysfunction*. The analogy of the powerhouse and the battery which I give in the chapter on Exercise (page 234) to explain the energy-producing function of the cell is relevant here. The mitochondria is the 'battery' in each cell which provides the body with rapidly-releasing energy. In a healthy person, the battery is recharged more or less immediately, but researchers suspect that in ME patients, this mechanism may be faulty. Delayed or impeded recharging of cellular energy could damage the cell structure and the mitochondria.

EXERCISE CAN EXACERBATE ME

These studies go a long way towards explaining a major problem experienced by ME sufferers – that associated with physical activity. A typical pattern is one where a person may have rested for a few hours, felt a bit better so decided to go for a walk, do some housework, pick up the weekly shopping, etc. (all reasonable and normal activities in the healthy and fit) but then, as a result of their efforts, felt worse; aching, tired and suffering from an increase in 'poisoned', flu-like symptoms. This time, they need to rest for longer. Then they may overdo things again but, as a result, will feel far worse for longer still . . . and so it goes on. Their 'recharge' facility is not functioning as it should and is taking an ever-increasing amount of time to recover.

WHO SUFFERS?

ME can affect anyone at any age, all races and both genders – from toddlers to octogenarians – but there do appear to be certain groups who are more at risk. Research shows that the 20s, 30s and 40s age groups are most susceptible, that women are twice as likely to go down as men.

An increasing number of young children and teenagers are now being diagnosed; recent surveys suggest that upwards of 12,000 may be affected in the UK alone. When symptoms first manifest, laziness or 'school phobia' are often blamed. Sadly, allegedly grown-up people have a nasty habit of ignoring their children. We pretend to listen but often don't hear. ME certainly seems to bring the cynical doubters out of the woodwork!

I find it particularly interesting that ME also appears to afflict the carers in our society, the majority of whom are women. That's not to say that all carers go down with ME but that they may be a more susceptible group. Caring for someone else, as so many of us are aware, can be exhausting and debilitating. It can also be a lonely task; when a carer feels unwell, how many complain? They feel a duty, priority and, often, a genuine feeling of not wanting to let down the person in their care. To complain is to whinge when someone else is worse off than you are? Right?

Wrong!

Here we go again, not taking care of ourselves.

It's perfectly possible that a carer's immunity is more susceptible to attack by an opportunist virus by the very fact that they are overtired, run down, possibly not eating as well as they should, probably sleeping with one ear and one eye open to the needs of their charge, not getting proper rest and being permanently 'on call'. They may also be working in areas where viruses are more prevalent: hospitals, nursing homes, etc.

Teachers are another 'at risk' group, being exposed to a wide range of circulating viruses in the classroom. And like the carers, teachers are often under considerable stress. As we have seen on pages 9–54, stress can be a detrimental factor in any illness, especially where immunity is already compromised.

IS THERE A CANDIDA CONNECTION?

A significant number of practitioners and patients believe that candida albicans is a common aggravator of ME and CFS. Others are less convinced and think the syndrome highly overrated. Candida is present in everyone, they argue. In addition, not everyone with candidiasis will suffer with ME; nor will every ME sufferer be plagued by candida.

WHAT IS CANDIDA?

Candida albicans is a yeast which moves into our inner tubes not long after we are born. Where good health and homoeostatic balance is maintained, the yeast lives in harmony with other natural inhabitants in the gut. Unfortunately, there are many instances where the candida can proliferate and change from its relatively harmless structure into an invasive fungus which penetrates the membrane between the digestive system and the bloodstream. Once the gut wall has been breached and made 'leaky', unwelcome molecules and toxic substances can pass easily into the blood system, alerting the immune system to invasion. If left untreated, the immunity soon becomes overworked and then weakened, increasing the risk of allergic reactions to food, chemicals and other environmental agents.

ANTI-CANDIDA DIETS – ARE THEY WORTHWHILE?

There is no doubt that strict anti-candida therapy has proven helpful to a significant number of ME sufferers. However, the suggestion has been made that anti-candida diets work only because they also eliminate the majority of common food allergens. This latter view may go some way to explain why the Food Combining Diet has worked well as an anti-candida treatment for so many people whereas an overly restricted diet can have a counterproductive effect. Too little variety can lead to a reduced number of nutrients and consequent malnutrition. Candida just adores to run riot in a nutrient-deficient system.

GENTLY DOES IT

My own experience with patients – and that of colleagues – has been that natural anti-fungal supplements such as mycopryl, garlic and acidophilus, together with perma-trol (for leaky gut syndrome), would appear to be particularly effective when used in conjunction with *gentle* dietary change and the elimination of only half a dozen or so of the most troublesome foods. Aggressive treatment with inflexible diet can be difficult to stick to and boring to follow. Such regimes tend to find favour because they can bring about startling results in the early stages – although long-term benefits are not always maintained. They may work for a stoical few but are not recommended for long-term use; for the majority, such restriction could be potentially damaging, both physi-cally and psychologically.

If you are intending to try a vigorous anti-candida diet, please obtain professional advice before you begin and make sure that you use immune-boosting and anti-fungal supplements in accordance with your practitioner's recommendations. Promise. This is important.

LET'S GET POSITIVE

Don't give up. The situation is far from hopeless. Gaining official recognition is a big step forward. Research into ME and associated illnesses is ongoing and we understand more about this condition than ever before.

ORTHODOX ACCEPTANCE

A National ME Task Force, set up in 1994, agrees that the condition is widespread, that there is a significant lack of support from doctors, no organized care for sufferers and a need for further high quality research. The fact that the Task Force has been organized by senior medics bodes well for ME and CFS sufferers although, of course, it is not saying anything new. **Action for ME** has been campaigning along these lines for a number of years.

DOCTORS SUFFER

Progress may also come from the fact that a number of doctors have, themselves, been stricken with the disease. It's a sad but true fact of life that we often don't see the other person's point of view until we are affected directly with the same problem!

THE GOOD NEWS

An increasing number of practitioners see ME not only as treatable but as curable. I have worked with many (suspected and confirmed) cases of ME and find that those patients who take an active part in their treatment demonstrate the greatest chance of recovery. There are a number of different therapies which seem particularly helpful and, also, a great deal that sufferers and helpers can do to encourage healing and mending.

With so much valuable information on ME and related conditions this chapter could turn, all too easily, into a book all on its own but space won't allow. It's a comfort to know that the search for causes and cures doesn't stop; every time a new paper is published, we take a step nearer to solving the ME puzzle. Whilst preparing this chapter, I pored over mountains of research material and, after several months, actually ran out of storage space. It was, for me, an absolutely fascinating – almost addictive – experience. The more I read, the more I wanted to learn.

I hope that the information given in other sections of *All Day Energy* and, also, that which follows will be useful. The chapters on Energy and the Environment (page 125), Stress (page 9), Sleep (page 89), Eating for Energy (Food and Supplements, page 307) should be of particular interest to ME sufferers.

1. One of the most important steps on your road to recovery is to find a sympathetic and understanding GP. You will need him or her to carry out a range of tests to confirm or eliminate ME from your diagnosis. An interested and conscientious doctor will do a full examination, including blood profile, urine and stool analysis. **Action for ME and Chronic Fatigue** is the best place to find help on how to work with your doctor *for your benefit* and how to change doctors if the one you have isn't helping you. If you do decide to change GPs, it can be a comfort to know that you don't have to give any notice or explanation to your present GP about the proposed change.

2. **Action for ME and Chronic Fatigue.** Their information pack contains useful addresses, recommended reading, help and advice on how to get a diagnosis, how to approach your GP, what to do if you are stonewalled, what tests, treatments and services are available and how to take an active part in your recovery. Highly recommended, of inestimable value for sufferers and essential assistance for families, carers, doctors and therapists.

Action for ME members receive the journal *InterAction*.

The ME Association may also be able to provide information. For details of telephone helplines and addresses for both these organizations, see Products and Services, page 351.

3.   Order *Guide to Candida and ME – possible causes and likely treatments* from the WDDTY organization (stands for *What Doctors Don't Tell You*). Essential and inexpensive reading. (See Recommended Reading, page 340).

4.   Top of the list of the most helpful treatments for ME is REST, REST, REST. It can be difficult for ME sufferers to accept the need for frequent rest and relaxation because they are so often active people who want to get on with life. It has to be appreciated, however, that overactivity and excessive physical exercise are two of the major causes of worsening ME symptoms.

5.   Tissue hypoxia (lack of oxygen) has been linked to Chronic Fatigue Syndrome and a consequent increase in muscle tenderness. One way of improving oxygen flow is to exercise but, unfortunately, strong aerobic activity usually makes ME symptoms worse. Deep breathing, however, helps to push more oxygen through the system without excessive physical exertion. The chapter on Exercise and Energy (page 219) contains some easy-to-follow breathing and stretching exercises which are gentle enough for anyone with ME or Chronic Fatigue symptoms to follow.

Hyperventilation is another common feature of the condition. Again, deep breathing exercises – used in conjunction with adequate rest and a modified diet and supplement programme – are good starting points.

6.   If you are still thinking of giving up, take heart from

this. One former patient who first approached me for help in 1992, wrote to me in the summer of 1994:

> It is now a couple of years since I came to consult your opinion on ME and diet. I am so glad that I had such faith and perservered. I have no craving whatsoever for chocolates or junk food. I have overcome all my food allergies except the one related to cow's milk (which I now avoid) . . . it seems more than certain that the good news is due to food combining.

This is a view commonly expressed. Food combining certainly does seem to be helpful in the treatment of a number of conditions and has been especially beneficial in enhancing energy levels, overcoming digestive and bowel disorders and, in turn, dealing with food allergies. More information appears on pages 273–279.

7. Seek out a qualified practitioner who is familiar with nutritional therapy. Before you book an appointment, however, ask about their success rates in treating ME, Chronic Fatigue Syndrome and Candida. Are they willing to put you in touch with other patients who are benefiting from their treatment? This is an important area. Dietary management has been shown to help around three-quarters of ME sufferers. Pages 257–292 should help with some food ideas too.

8. Make sure your diet is not too restricted and don't cut down too far on protein. Insufficient protein lowers vitality.

9. Up your intake of fresh fruits and vegetables and try to keep your diet as 'clean' as possible. Take whatever steps you can to avoid factory farmed meat and poultry, battery eggs and non-organic produce. This makes good

health sense for anyone but could be vital for anyone suffering from ME or CFS. There is increasing concern among a number of experts that the drug residues and chemicals which have become so much a part of commercial food production may be implicated in diseases involving the nervous system. Support the Farm Animal Network and Compassion in World Farming organizations and contact The Soil Association for details of suppliers of organic produce in your area (see Products and Services – page 346).

No-one is likely to be able to stay completely clear of crop sprays, food additives and other chemicals all the time but it's worth making the effort to pass by the prepackaged, the processed and the preserved where there are fresh and unadulterated alternatives, especially if your health depends upon it.

10. Always have breakfast but be careful in your choices. The so-called healthy start to the day of juice, toast, cereal and tea or coffee may seem a good option because it is low in fat and low in protein. But watch out! This veritable feast of potential allergens can be anathema to an already sensitive system. Temperamental digestion? Irritable bowel? Suspected allergies? If that's you, then orange juice, wheat, cow's milk and caffeine are to be avoided. Definite outsiders in the usable energy department. Trust me!!!!!

An additional complaint of the string and sawdust breakfast (apart from the fact that it tastes like string and sawdust) is that it doesn't sustain the appetite for very long. Come mid-morning, the abdomen may bloat but the stomach is empty. Devotees of this 'continental con' may find themselves gnawing with hunger and checking out the chocolate at break time. A light protein-based breakfast is often a better option for anyone suffering from fatigue.

11.   To get you started – and while you are collating information and looking for a helpful practitioner – these are the foods that you should avoid: Sugar, chocolate, coffee, yeast, bread, wheat-based breakfast cereals, hydrogenated spreads, 'ready' meals, cow's milk and related products, beef and pork. Eat unadulterated fresh foods which you prepare from basics at home, choose organic produce whenever possible and keep packeted, processed food to an absolute minimum.

12.   Treat yourself to a regular aromatherapy massage, a gentle but effective 'exercise' which you don't have to do yourself. Massage also helps to de-stress and relax you – and to push a bit more of that valuable oxygen around your aching muscles.

13.   Try to remove as many potential toxins from your living, working and sleeping environment as possible. The chapter on Energy and the Environment (page 125) is an essential read for anyone with chronic fatigue.

14.   Worth mentioning is the experience of some practitioners that a good quality Vitamin B Complex daily (or a Multivitamin/Mineral Complex which contains reasonable doses of the major B vitamins) has been helpful in relieving chronic fatigue. This is unlikely to be effective in isolation but can be a useful 'back-up' to other treatments, particularly an improved diet. Avoid any products labelled B vitamin 'compound', however. They may be cheaper but some brands have caused what appear to be allergic reactions, cramps and indigestion. Such symptoms could mean that the product is not well absorbed,

could be taxing on the liver and using up unnecessary energy. People suffering from ME, food allergies or other digestive problems, would be wise to steer clear of any Vitamin B combinations which contain yeast.

15.   Obtain as much information as possible about the vitamin, mineral and other supplements which have been shown to be helpful in relieving ME (and Candida) symptoms. The recommended reading at the beginning of this section (pages 205 and 206) and on page 340 will guide you. If you have no-one to advise you just at the moment, you could still try out this basic programme and then change or modify it once you have practitioner support: With food, take –

EITHER	4 to 6 evening primrose oil capsules daily
OR	2 GLA capsules daily
PLUS	1 garlic capsule or tablet daily
	1 multivitamin/mineral complex daily
AND	2 grams vitamin C complex (as magnesium ascorbate) daily

Make sure your multivitamin/mineral contains magnesium, selenium, chromium and zinc.

The mineral magnesium has been shown in studies to be beneficial to some ME patients and it may be worthwhile taking extra amounts. Talk to your practitioner about this. Injections may be available (**Action for ME** has details); otherwise, magnesium in capsule form could be an alternative. When it comes to any kind of supplement, good general advice is to buy the best that you can afford. Although it doesn't always follow, my experience has been that ingredients in some of the cheaper products have made symptoms worse and may do nothing more than add to the toxic overload. Magnesium oxide, for example, has been known to cause stomach pain and diarrhoea. I have found the more expensive magnesium fumarate, magnesium phosphoserine, magnesium taurate and magnesium EAP all helpful in reducing muscle pain, spasm and tenderness and I have not come across any adverse reactions. Check the label and ask your practitioner and supplier if you are in any doubt about what kind of magnesium you are taking.

16.   Ginkgo biloba and other flavonoids – such as bilberry and beetroot extract – have been studied as possible remedies for tissue hypoxia (oxygen starvation) and may offer additional protection. Ginkgo has been shown to improve circulation and memory recall. More information on this is in the Supplements for Energy section on page 308.

17.   See a chiropractor or osteopath and get your bones checked. Spinal misalignment can increase muscle spasm, pain and fatigue. A regular, twice yearly once-over is a good investment. See Products and Services (page 352) for details of how to find a practitioner.

18.   Drink plenty of water. I make no apologies for repeating this point. Yes, yes. Nag, nag, nag. ME patients should aim for around two litres of water (preferably filtered) per day to reduce the risk of toxins building up in the system and to keep the lymphatic system, liver, bowels, kidneys and skin as healthy as possible.

19.   Talk to your GP about a course of Vitamin B_{12} injections. Whilst some research shows B_{12} has not been beneficial, other work suggests that it can be a helpful tonic. Treatment is safe and cost is low. Worth trying. If

injections are not available to you, page 355 has details of where to obtain a course of quality tablets. More information on this on page 315.

20.   Around 40 per cent of sufferers in one survey said that herbal medicine has helped to relieve symptoms. A properly tailored programme can improve the function of the lymphatic and nervous systems, the liver, kidneys and adrenals, act as a blood tonic and generally rebalance the body. However, herbal medicines need to be tailored to individual requirements. Chinese medical herbalists would first carry out a full examination before recommending treatment including tongue and pulse examination. Don't self-medicate herbal treatments. Make the effort to obtain professional advice and consult a qualified therapist. The section on page 352 carries details.

21.   The prevalence of gut disorders in ME sufferers is worth special mention and is a point you should discuss with your practitioner. Malabsorption syndrome, which increases the risk of nutrient deficiency, is often associated with bacterial fermentation of the colon, insufficient pancreatic enzymes and low levels of stomach acid. Not surprisingly, food intolerance, flatulence, bloating, general digestive discomfort and bowel disorders are common symptoms but are not always related to candida albicans. Tests and treatments are available. (See Products and Services.)

22.   Take a course of probiotic supplements to help restore damaged gut flora, improve bowel function and reduce bloating. My husband Ralph takes these every day and has found them to be particularly helpful in relieving the digestive discomforts caused by having had his

stomach removed. Over the years, he has become something of a connoisseur of probiotic products and has tried several brands. Disappointingly, however, only a handful of brands seem to be effective. More information on page 355.

23.   Use fresh garlic in your cooking and take a daily capsule or tablet of top quality garlic, shown to be especially helpful in the treatment of candidiasis and ME related symptoms. (Bear in mind that the completely deodorized garlic may not be so effective.) See Nutrients for Energy (page 307) for more information.

24.   If you are getting nowhere with your treatment, consider the possibility of intestinal parasites, such as giardia. Don't freak out; it's very common. A diligent doctor will check for this familiar gut dweller and treat accordingly. Whilst a short course of antibiotics is a commonly used treatment for the condition, these drugs are not recommended where there is ME, chronic fatigue or candida, *unless absolutely necessary*. Indeed, some experts are convinced that one or all of these conditions may be triggered by over-enthusiastic antibiotic exposure.

Supplements based on grapefruit seed extract, artemesia annua, echinacea and garlic have been shown to be very effective and may be a safer bet in the long term. Homoeopathic Cina 6C or Teucrium 6C are also well worth trying. Information can be found in Products and Services – page 355.

25.   Along with antibiotics, tranquillizers and steroid drugs were named as medications used in the treatment of ME which, according to a large group of surveyed patients, were actually *detrimental* to their condition. If these are prescribed for you, ask lots of questions and find

out if they are absolutely necessary. For more information on drugs and their side effects, contact WDDTY; details can be found on page 340.

My thanks must go to Action for ME and Chronic Fatigue for the help they have provided. Also to Nick Hall, Division of Psychoimmunology, TGH Psychiatry Center USF, Tampa, Florida.

SOURCES OF REFERENCE:

Cox I M, Campbell M J & Dowson D. Red blood cell magnesium and chronic fatigue syndrome. *Lancet* 1991;337:757–60.

Lee M M. Chronic Fatigue Syndrome – The Conundrum, The Cure. *Blackmores Communicator* 1991; issue 4, volume 5.

Rosen H, Blumenthal A & Agersborg H. Effects of the potassium and magnesium salts of aspartic acid on metabolic exhaustion. *Journal of Pharmaceutical Science* 1962;51:592.

Simpson L. Myalgic Encephalomyelitis. *Journal of the Royal Society of Medicine* October 1993 p. 633.

Schaffler V & Reeh P. Double-blind study of the hypoxia protective effect of a standardized ginkgo biloba preparation after repeated administration in healthy volunteers. *Arzneim-Forsch* 1985;35:1283–6.

Ryan C F. Letter to *Journal of Orthomolecular Medicine* 1989;4[4]:233–4.

Shafran S D et al. Chronic Fatigue Syndrome. *American*

Journal of Medicine 1991;90:730–40.

Costa D C. The study of the blood flow through the brainstems of people with ME, depressed patients and controls. Presentation at The Institute of Nuclear Medicine, University College London Medical School; 30 March 1994.

Jones J F, Ray C G, Minnich L L et al. Evidence for active Epstein-Barr virus infection in patients with persistent, unexplained illnesses: elevated anti-early antigen antibodies. *Annals of Internal Medicine* 1985;102:1–7.

Calder B D, Warnock P J, McCartney R A, Bell E J. Coxsackie B viruses and the post-viral syndrome: a prospective study in general practice. *Journal of the Royal College of General Practitioners* 1987;37:11–14.

Morriss R et al. Abnormalities of Sleep in Patients with Chronic Fatigue Syndrome. *British Medical Journal* 1993;306:1161–4.

Fatigue Chemical Identified. Report in *Blackmores Communicator* 1994;2(8):2.

Krupp L B et al. Sleep Disturbance in Chronic Fatigue Syndrome. *Journal of Psychosomatic Research* 1993;37(4):325–31.

Dunstan R H et al. Chronic Fatigue Syndrome: A Unirary Biomarker. Paper presented at International CFS Meeting. Dublin, May 1994.

Ellis F R & Nasser S. A pilot study of Vitamin B_{12} in the treatment of tiredness. *British Journal of Nutrition* 1973;30:277–83.

Straus S E, Tosato G, Armstrong G et al. Persisting illness and fatigue in adults with evidence of Epstein-Barr virus infection. *Annals of Internal Medicine* 1985; 102:7–16.

Steinbach T L et al. Treatment of CFIDS with Kutapressin [liver extract and by-product of Vitamin B12]. *Chronic Fatigue and Immune Dysfunction Journal* 1990; Spring/Summer issue: 25–30.

Holmes G P, Kaplan J E, Stewart J A et al. A cluster of patients with a chronic mononucleosis-like syndrome. Is Epstein-Barr virus the cause? *Journal of the American Medical Association* 1987;257:2297–302.

Eggar J et al. Magnesium for hyperventilation in Retts Syndrome. *Lancet* 1992;340:621–2.

Bell E J, McCartney R A, Riding M H. Coxsackie B viruses and myalgic encephalomyelitis. *Journal of the Royal Society of Medicine* 1988;81:329–31.

Ho-Yen D O et al. Natural killer cells and the post viral fatigue syndrome. *Scandinavian Journal of Infectious Diseases* 1991;23:711–716.

Costa D C et al. Brain stem hypoperfusion in patients with myalgic encephalomyelitis – chronic fatigue syndrome. *European Journal of Nuclear Medicine* 1992; 19[8]:733.

Behan W M H et al. Mitochondrial abnormalities in postviral fatigue syndrome. *Acta Neuropathologica* 1991; 83:61–5.

Riley M S et al. Aerobic work capacity in patients with chronic fatigue syndrome. *British Medical Journal* 1990; 301:953–6.

Wood C. Diurnal changes in perception of energy and mood. *Journal of the Royal Society of Medicine* 1992; 85:191–4.

Wood C. Mood change and perceptions of vitality: a comparison of the effects of relaxation, visualization and yoga. *Journal of the Royal Society of Medicine* 1993;86:254–8.

Demitrack M A et al. Evidence for impaired activation of the hypothalmic-pituitary-adrenal axis in patients with chronic fatigue syndrome. *Journal of Clinical Endocrinology and Metabolism* 1991;73(6):1224–34.

An Alternative to Psychiatry by Tuula Tuorma, The Book Guild, 1991.

9

Exercise for Energy

'Those who think they have not time for bodily exercise will sooner or later have to find time for illness.'

Edward Stanley, Earl of Derby (1826–93)
British Statesman

There is no doubt about it; exercise can improve the quality of your life and your health. But that means choosing the correct level of exercise attuned to your personal preference and individual requirements. Being forced into an exercise routine that you dislike intensely and which makes you feel anything less than rejuvenated is definitely not the right choice.

For some, the very word 'exercise' is immoral. It was Henry Ford who was supposed to have said 'Exercise is bunk. If you are healthy you don't need it. If you are sick, you shouldn't take it.' Presumably, he had car sales in mind. At around the same time, his views were confirmed by the American humorist, Ring Lardner Jnr, whose only exercise, he boasted, was taking collar studs out of one shirt and putting them into another.

Unfortunately, physical activity has, for many people, an image of pain and strain rather than pleasure and satisfaction. We all hear stories about the sports injury, the accident at the aerobics class or the jogger who died suddenly from a heart attack. You could get the idea that anything more vigorous than a snail's pace is bad news and should be avoided.

For out of shape individuals, moving furniture instead of collar studs, shovelling snow, running races or launching into heavy workout sessions – when they haven't done any exercise all year – is asking for trouble. In fact, because *sudden* activity in the unfit can block the flow of blood to the heart, researchers estimate the risk of a heart attack to be six times (!) more likely. That's why anyone who is new to exercise but wants to 'give it a go', should get a medical check-up before they begin any fitness programme.

If you are moderately and sensibly active, however, your risk is minimal. Indeed, the benefits of regular movement are legion. It strengthens the immunity, reduces the risk of brittle bone disease, improves circulation and the flow of oxygen to the cells, helps balance cholesterol and blood pressure, relieves depression and anxiety and lessens the risk of heart disease. And that's just for starters. A couple of things in particular that should be of interest to almost everyone are – point one – that regular physical activity reduces the effects of ageing and – a very important point two – **exercise equals energy.**

But does exercise equal weight loss?
At the right level, in conjunction with other healthy activities – such as eating right – yes. If you are overweight to begin with, then quality Calories and quality exercise are a powerful combination. However, if you are exercising because you've heard that it's the *only* way to lose weight, have a care! It's helpful, of course. But not if your diet is a load of junk or you are unfit or undernourished.

Take the 'you never see any fat postmen' stuff with a

pinch of salt. We've all seen overweight posties. Remarks like that prove nothing. They are thrown out to persuade you that because postmen supposedly get lots of exercise, then exercise must be the primary answer to all weight problems. Not for every postman, it isn't. Not for you, either. Nor does it follow, necessarily, that if you run like a greyhound, you will automatically end up being built like a greyhound (dog, not bus!). You could end up broken down and out of fuel if you don't take care.

USE IT OR LOSE IT!

Exercise is about strength, endurance, flexibility, fitness, balance and co-ordination. All these vital factors are interlinked and are the benefits which accrue from properly planned, *regularly taken* activity. 'Regular' is a key word here. The oft-used phrase 'use it or lose it' really does apply to exercise. Improvements will be maintained only with commitment.

TIRED OR ELATED?

Any form of exercise can be tiring if you exceed your present fitness level. Exercise programmes should be enjoyable. If they're not, either you are doing the wrong one or doing it the wrong way. On completion of any routine, you should feel good. If you don't sleep well or if you are tired and achy the next day, then you may have done too much – or not have prepared your body properly. All the more reason to start with 'little and often' exercises to see how you go!

This book is, primarily, about energy, not about specific exercise and so I am *not* going to fill it with illustrations of incredibly fit workout freaks doing unattainable things that make everyone else feel inadequate. There is nothing worse than an over-enthusiastic physical jerk with 'abs' like steel who thinks that his or her routine is the only one that the rest of the world should follow. Happily, they are in a minority but they do exist and have been especially prominent in a few of the videos of recent years! The damage that can be – and has been – caused by super-zealous muscle mechanics underlines the vital importance of training with qualified teachers who have empathy with *your* needs.

TAKE IT E-A-S-Y!

I wouldn't dream of encouraging you to take up exercise from instructions in a book, simply because I have no idea of your present fitness level. What I have done, with the help of some talented experts, is include some *humane* exercises which involve more in the way of stretching, breathing, stress relief and relaxation than sweaty lurching, leaping or stepping. The gentle approach is the best way to *begin* your joyful journey on the road to improved energy and fitness.

I'll never forget how much I laughed at Susan Powter's description of her first visit to an aerobics class. The 'not very bright' instructor was yelling and screaming commands at her class. The then out-of-breath, eighteen and a half stone (and very unfit) Susan wanted to know how she was supposed to be able to jump, breathe, smile and hold 'abs in' all at the same time. Her book, *Stop the Insanity*, is recommended reading for anyone who thinks they are too far down the road to change – or has had a basinful of being 'put down' by *alleged* experts – and is worth it for the exercise you'll get laughing at her wonderful characterizations.

PLAN AHEAD

Exercise programmes should be tailored for the individual and should take account of your health history and your present fitness level. If you are fed up with aerobics classes which give the impression of 'Fit people only beyond this point', then get help from real experts who understand that everyone has individual requirements and who appreciate the value of individual assessment and attention.

Before you launch into classes of any kind, check out the qualifications of your instructor-to-be. At the time of writing, UK based teachers may not have professional indemnity insurance unless they sport the letters RSA (Royal Society of Arts) or NVQ (National Vocational Qualification). Fitness professionals who have trained with PEA (Physical Education Association) or YMCA will be similarly qualified. However, letters and names of associations do change, so don't be afraid to check out the information you've been given.

THE EXERCISE ASSOCIATION

The Exercise Association, who I found to be very helpful,

will advise on current training standards and also provide details of qualified instructors in your local area. They can also point you in the right direction for equipment, clothing, videos and national fitness events. You'll find their address, together with other sources of information, on page 348.

CHOOSE THE EXERCISE WHICH FEELS RIGHT FOR YOU

Consider every kind of exercise before you make a decision. Swimming, keep-fit classes, cycling (moving or stationary), dancing, sensible weight training, aerobics, rebounding, t'ai chi, yoga – even simple stretching exercises – are all worth investigating. If nothing else, brisk walking for half an hour a day should help to keep you in shape as long as you are not doing it in company with articulated trucks and traffic smog. Having said that, using your feet instead of the bus is still worthwhile exercise, but do avoid traffic fumes for at least part of your route, and wear the correct footwear.

WALK ON

Sorry to sound like a school ma'am but if you choose walking, please wear sensible footwear! Teetering along in platforms or stilettos not only looks ridiculous but is also likely to damage your back and destroy your posture. If you go in for longer hikes, then invest in a pair of good walking shoes and a backpack or rucksack for the essential bits and pieces. No-one can exercise properly when carrying a handbag or briefcase!

Arms should be relaxed and swinging when you are walking; thumbs turned slightly outwards and elbows in. If you can't get to a suitable area (i.e. are hemmed in by main roads, have no green space nearby, etc.), then use the stairs. Alternate by walking up and down on flat feet and then doing it again on your toes. Feel the muscles working.

BE PREPARED

Warming up and winding down movements are as important as the exercise session itself but, even here, you could be increasing the risk of injury if you don't know what you're about. A couple of private lessons with a qualified fitness instructor could be worth its weight in weights and may save you from injury later on.

IN FOR A STRETCH

S-t-r-e-t-c-h-i-n-g, both before and after exercise, improves joint mobility, stability, posture and balance. It also increases the flow of blood to the muscles, helping them to flex and relax and protecting them from damage. Observe animals, particularly cats, and see how they stretch.

When muscles are tight, the transport of oxygen and other vital nourishment will be restricted. In the same way that inadequate breathing can induce fatigue, lack of oxygen to muscle tissue can cause muscle fatigue. Knackered muscles won't be able to absorb the pounding force and impact which is bound to occur during aerobic exercise. If you have overdone it during a workout session, stretching *after* the event can reduce muscle soreness. Stretching also allows space for 'private time', a quiet period where mind and body can connect, while you are preparing to *power up* or *power off*.

It's never too late to start; indeed, stretching becomes all the more important as we age, helping to keep us mobile. Try the stretching exercises which begin on page 249. When you first attempt them, they will take a little longer but, once mastered, will take about 2 minutes (!) a day. No excuses *here* that exercise is time-consuming!

Take care!

DON'T stretch:	If your body is chilled
or	If the room you are in is cold
DON'T stretch:	If you have any sprains or strains
	If you are injured in any way
or	If you are in pain

TAKE PROFESSIONAL ADVICE ON STRETCHING AND OTHER EXERCISES:

If you are pregnant

If you suffer with	osteoporosis
	a heart condition
	any arthritic or rheumatic condition

---

a back problem
hypermobility
fibromyalgia
chronic fatigue syndrome
or   ME
      if you have limited range of
      movement due to disability or
      immobility
or   if you have recently had any
      kind of surgery or are waiting
      for an operation

How to s-t-r-e-t-c-h
*** Relax before stretching.
*** Never stretch cold muscles.
*** Walk up and down on the spot for a couple of
    minutes to warm up.
*** Stretch warmed muscles before and after
    activity.
*** Don't force the movement.
*** Work within your own limits.
*** Do your stretches every day even if you are not
    intending to do a full exercise programme.
*** Learn to balance each stretch with a corre-
    sponding muscle group, i.e. front of thigh
    (quadriceps) and back of thigh (hamstrings).
*** Don't stretch to the point of pain.

*** If it hurts before you begin, then DON'T do it.
*** If it hurts during the stretch, then STOP!
*** Don't workout on a completely empty stomach. If your blood glucose levels are low, you won't have the stamina and could increase the risk of reactive hypoglycaemia.
*** But don't exercise *immediately* after a meal either, unless you fancy a fit of indigestion. An hour or two – no more – is about right between food and exercise.
*** Check that the person advising you is properly qualified.
*** For further information, see Products and Services page 348.

If you jog or walk out of doors, get street smart: These days, the pollution thrown up by road vehicles makes a nonsense of jogging or walking near main traffic thoroughfares. Breathe in all those toxic fumes and it's a fair bet your health could suffer more than if you didn't exercise at all! The down side is that you may be swapping security for better air quality. Being on guard isn't paranoid, it's simply sensible:
*** Try to avoid going out at dawn or dusk, but if you do, wear something bright – or white – to enable motorists to see you clearly.

*** Carry a personal alarm in your hand or on your belt and know how to activate it.

*** If you wear a bum bag or fanny pack, make sure it's a slim one you can tuck out of sight under your shirt.

*** Leave your radio/tape at home and don't wear headphones. You may not hear a stranger approaching.

*** If possible, find a friend or partner to share your exercise sessions with you.

*** Vary your route.

*** Wear a top which shouts 'tough, keep off'; for example, the name of your local karate club or fitness centre.

*** Tuck long hair into a hat or cap.

*** If you jog with the dog, call him (or her!) 'Killer' when you're out. Reserve 'Fifi' or 'Cuddles' for home use only!

*** Look as if you mean business. Move confidently.

*** Be safety conscious without looking nervous. It's worth assuming that every stranger is suspect especially if you are out alone.

*** If you are concerned that someone may be following you, get yourself to an area where there are more people.

*** Don't wear jewellery and keep your watch out of sight.

*** If someone asks the time, you don't have it.

*** In the unlikely event of your being

approached, be firm, don't lower your gaze (it can make you seem submissive), keep moving and don't be afraid to make a lot of noise. Use a commanding tone, not a pleading one. Show that you are in control. Research indicates that potential attackers are anxious, on edge and far more likely to give up on someone who is dominating, decisive and making a hell of a din.

No amount of exercising is going to be totally beneficial if you don't, first, learn how to B-R-E-A-T-H-E. To ancient traditions, it is breathing rather than eating which brings energy to the body. That's not to say that we should give up food, of course, but rather that 'power' will not be channelled into the system without the slow, rhythmical intake of air. Try breathing without eating and the human frame can survive for long periods of time. Try eating without breathing and you may find yourself in difficulty.

Learning to breathe properly and efficiently is one of the best ways of channelling new energy into the body. Trouble is, most of us never give our breathing a second thought — it's something which just happens. Why waste time worrying about a reaction which is automatic anyway? As long as we breathe somehow, that's good enough isn't it?

That depends, I guess, on what you want out of life.

Opting for a less than optimum oxygen intake can make you feel sluggish, listless and generally under par. Observe what happens to the breath when we are upset or angry, for example. It becomes short, tight and strained. 'A sharp intake of breath' is a common stress reaction; some people respond to a traumatic situation by stopping breathing altogether. The body's response to lack of air is one of the reasons we resort to sighing when we are upset; it's a deep breath followed by a long exhalation. Those who are under constant pressure are inclined to sigh a great deal. If you recognize yourself here, the exercises which follow could be particularly beneficial.

THE AIR THAT WE BREATHE

All day energy is far less likely if your breathing isn't deep enough. Cutting down on oxygen cuts down on stamina, reduces resistance to stress and increases the risk of illness. Strong, deep and full breathing sends *life* flowing through to the deepest recesses of the body and brain, activating, energizing and calming all at the same time. Indian yoga also teaches that all the body's ailments are, for better or for worse, under the control of the mind and the emotions, and by enhancing the quality and depth of the breathing we can create an internal environment which is hostile to disease.

GOOD GAS!

A simple analogy which explains the vital connection between breathing and energy production is the internal combustion engine in your car. Neither the body nor the car can function without fuel. But to make that fuel supply work, something else is required.

Oxygen, O_2.

The way in which it works is nothing short of breathtaking!

Inlet, compression, power, exhaust is the process by which petroleum gases are burnt and waste products discharged from a road vehicle. Your car engine 'inhales' oxygen from outside the vehicle which then reacts with the fuel to produce energy in order to drive the machine along. This reaction produces waste gases which are expelled via the exhaust system.

In a very similar way, you draw air from outside the body into the lungs. The body needs that oxygen to metabolize food and convert it into energy. The *inlet* is the breathing in of oxygen which is then pushed (the *compression*) via the bloodstream through tiny blood vessels (the capillaries) and into the cells. In every cell are microscopic powerhouses called mitochondria which use oxygen to burn whatever kind of food (fuel) that particular cell happens to need, be it glucose, fat or protein.

Poor quality breathing means that the transport of life-giving O_2 via the bloodstream to the 'powerhouse' is reduced. We are not talking about the odd cell or two being affected; there are billions of cells beavering away in your system. They all need oxygen to live. If they don't produce any energy, neither do you. If they don't live, neither do you.

The cellular system also needs to keep the garbage disposal (the *exhaust*) working efficiently. In simple terms, waste products (i.e. carbon dioxide) can't be discharged from the cells and back to the lungs for excretion if sufficient oxygen doesn't reach the cells in the first place.

RECHARGE!

In very simple terms, you could picture the mitochondria (the powerhouse) in each cell as a battery. When you take in oxygen, the battery is recharged. As energy is released from the cell, the charge runs down until it is boosted again by more oxygen.

When you light a fire, you use fuel (coal, gas or logs, for example) and air to produce heat and flame (energy) in much the same way that the body burns its fuel (in this case from food) to produce energy. If you prevent air reaching the source of the flame, the fire will suffocate – just as your system would without oxygen. In addition, if the fire continues to burn but the waste cannot escape (through the chimney), then the building will be filled with toxic smoke. If you didn't clean out the grate regularly, the next fire wouldn't light or burn as brightly.

The body reacts in a similar way.

Reduced oxygen = reduced energy = a build-up of toxic waste = sluggishness = eventual breakdown.

In other words, no spark, no fire, no energy, no life!

PREVENTION IS BETTER THAN CURE

If your car breaks down, you might think of booking it in for a service or, in an emergency, calling your motoring rescue organization. Unfortunately, humans seem to think that they can run their bodies on poor quality fuel with little or no oxygen and little or no maintenance. When something goes wrong (whether it's a house filled with smoke, a car which won't start or a sick body), it's usually the emergency services who are called in to sort out the mess.

So, please, breathe more deeply. Become a chain breather – do it all the time. Your health depends on it.

TAKEN FOR GRANTED

There's an old Jewish proverb which goes: 'First you're born, then you die. Life's a bitch!' Breathing is the first and last thing we do in life but what happens in between? Total unawareness until something goes wrong! It's true that *breathing properly* is something we definitely don't do enough of. For example, when did you last move your lungs, those two huge air exchangers inside your rib cage? People who don't breathe deeply enough still survive because they do take in some air and expel some carbon dioxide. Unfortunately, they don't use their lungs to anything like full capacity. It's doubtful that the lower sections of the lung have seen oxygen for decades!

So, although you are almost certainly breathing (otherwise you wouldn't be reading this!), it may not be enough for your own long-term good.

A LEGACY FROM CHILDHOOD?

For some of us, breathing only into the upper chest was something instilled into us from childhood. 'Shoulders back, chest out, don't slouch' were the orders issued by parents and teachers with parade ground mentality. These very actions tighten and restrict most of the breathing apparatus, especially the ribs, the diaphragm and abdominal muscles. Try it yourself and see how difficult it becomes to breathe properly. In a similar way, wearing restrictive clothing such as boned corsets and tight bodices caused Victorian and Edwardian ladies to suffer from 'the vapours'.

Low energy levels, dizziness, fatigue, tension in the shoulders and a pain in the neck (!) are common symptoms of restrained respiration. At my old school, fainting in assembly was blamed on the fact that the girls enjoyed being carried to Matron's room by the blond and athletic sports master. A much more likely explanation, though, was inadequate breathing coupled to tight clothing and lack of breakfast! No way to reduce stress and increase energy!

BREATHING HAS BEEN AROUND FOR QUITE A WHILE

The 'life force' so familiar to Eastern medicine is hardly, if ever, discussed by Western medics. The Chinese believe that if the 'life force' – called Chi or Qi or, in Indian medicine, Prana – is obstructed by poor living habits, inadequate breathing, stress, lack of exercise and insufficient nourishment, then vitality and inner strength also diminish. Correct breathing is an essential contributor to physical, mental, emotional and spiritual well-being.

THIS IS HOW YOUR BODY BREATHES

In an area of the brain called the medulla oblongata resides a respiratory regulator. This fellow organizes the nerve impulses to the apparatus which helps us to inhale and exhale. As we breathe in, the intercostal muscles (situated between each rib) raise the rib cage, the diaphragm moves downwards and the lungs inflate. Because the air pressure inside the lungs is then lower than that outside the body, air rushes in to take up the space. Oxygen is drawn into the body and pushed, again by muscular action, through the bloodstream to the tissues. As we breathe out, the ribs move down, the diaphragm relaxes upwards and the lungs deflate, forcing out the carbon dioxide waste – and water vapour, which is why you can make a window steam up if you breathe onto it.

PUTTING MATTERS RIGHT

The very first thing you need to do is to find out if you are a belly breather or a chest breather.

Put your right hand on your upper chest and the other on your abdomen. Breathe normally but pay particular attention to the hand which moves the most. If the left hand moves more than the right, you are a belly breather. If the right hand moves but the left hand doesn't, you are probably breathing too shallowly, only taking a small amount of air into the upper chest area.

Next, place a hand on either side of your rib cage (just like putting your hands on your hips only higher up). Then take a normal breath in (not a deep breath — just your own average inhalation). Did you feel your rib cage move out sideways, pushing your hands away from the body? If not, you are definitely not breathing completely or thoroughly enough.

BREATHING UNDER STRESS

Rapid breathing or hyperventilation is a common response to a stressful situation. For a short while, the level of carbon dioxide in the bloodstream is reduced and the body takes in more oxygen than it needs; the result can be tingling hands and feet, a numbness in the lips, dizziness, blurred vision, confused thinking and poor co-ordination. The simplest way to redress the balance (in a real emergency) is *said* to be to breathe into a paper bag (never use polythene or plastic of any kind). Hold the paper over your mouth and nose for ten normal breaths. The re-used carbon dioxide is believed to be helpful in stabilizing the breathing and returning the situation to normal. Remember, this is only for use as an emergency measure. Cupping the hands over the nose and mouth seems to have a similarly calming effect. Although very little CO_2 is likely to be trapped in this way, the action of touching the face with the hands can, of itself, be soothing.

Prolonged hyperventilation (shallow, rapid breathing) has been studied by specialists at Addenbrooke's Hospital in Cambridge and is now considered an extremely common disorder. Unfortunately, however, the symptoms which hyperventilation produces are all too often labelled 'all in the mind'. Symptoms can include weakness, anxiety, stress, fatigue, muscle cramps, twitchy limbs, sweats, bad dreams, insomnia, headaches and palpitations.

Although not applicable in every situation, over-breathers are more likely to be perfectionists who drive themselves too hard, are often meticulously tidy, prone to frustration, hide their emotions and hate being late. An absence of emotional comfort and support – and feelings of insecurity during the formative years – may lead to an adult becoming a stressed overbreather who may take in twenty to twenty-four breaths each minute. The normal average is sixteen to eighteen. A slow steady breather, especially someone who practises breathing exercises and/or does regular yoga, will inhale and exhale around twelve to fourteen times every sixty seconds.

BREATHING BENEFITS

The actual breathing part of the exercises in this chapter are vitally important in the restoration of energy. Although extremely valuable in their own right, it would appear, from research and from clinical experience, that relaxation and visualization alone may not be as beneficial as when accompanied by yoga breathing (pranayama). In one particular study, carried out by the Department of Experimental Psychology at Oxford University, physical and mental energy were assessed in a group of seventy-one volunteers. The yogic breathing and stretching had a markedly invigorating effect upon the perception of energy and mood.

There are other benefits too. A clinical trial published in the *Lancet* in June 1990, demonstrated that yogic breathing can reduce the symptoms of asthma. In the twenty-two patients who took part, all aspects of lung function improved to some degree. Another study, reported in the *Journal of Asthma*, demonstrated a significant improvement in lung function and exercise capacity in asthmatic children who learned yogic breathing techniques. Since deep breathing techniques such as these are known to reduce the production of histamine, they may also be valuable in helping people who suffer from allergies and hay fever.

KATHRYN'S BASIC BREATHING EXERCISE

If you find it difficult to achieve a deep breathing rhythm, try the following exercise which is designed to help you increase your oxygen intake and expel carbon dioxide wastes more efficiently. Don't put any pressure on yourself to 'do it right'; just follow the guidelines and the flow and movement of breath will come. Do the exercise twice a day, for example, first thing in the morning before you get up – to help focus your thoughts for the day – and last thing at night while you are waiting to go to sleep.

*** Lie down and make sure you are completely comfortable. Be as relaxed as possible. For extra support and easier breathing, you may like to place a pillow or rolled towel under your neck and knees or, alternatively, lie with knees bent and the feet flat.

*** Exhale slowly and completely. Remember that exhalation is the relaxing part of the breath.

*** Then, inhale freely (through the nose, not the mouth), allowing your abdomen to extend and the lower ribs expand forwards and sideways. Don't be tempted to 'over-inhale'. Breathe to comfortable limits. Do not strain.

*** Then breathe out as slowly as possible, through the nose.

*** Repeat the in-breath and the out-breath ten times. As you progress, you should find that the inhalation will deepen automatically and that the exhalation will lengthen.

*** If you find that you can take in only a small amount of air, don't be concerned. You may even find that your rib cage and abdominal area move hardly at all. This is a very common experience. Regular twice daily practice will help to increase breathing capacity.

*** During the exercises, keep the mouth gently closed and breathe in and out through the nose. Remember: DO NOT STRAIN. Breathe to comfortable limits.

BREATHE YOUR WAY TO ENERGY

With any of the following exercises, always try to find a quiet place where there will be no distractions. Take the telephone off the hook. If noise intrudes, picture a sound-proofed wall between you and the disturbance. Every time you become aware of noise, push it away behind the wall.

Work on creating a safe sanctuary, a mind refuge where you can go whenever you want to do any of the following exercises or you just need a few moments peace and quiet. Imagine a place where you feel safe, settled and secure.

These imaging and breathing exercises are relaxing but also energizing. Practised and used regularly, they really do help to lift lethargy, reduce tension and clarify the mental processes.

Try the following exercises and see which ones suit you best. Then practise those on a regular basis and call on them in emergencies too.

THE DO-ANYWHERE WIND DOWN

Sit comfortably (either at your desk, in an armchair, at the dining table, on the floor, even in the car as long as you are parked up safely).
Close your eyes.
Think through your whole body and make sure that you are as relaxed as you can be. Pay particular attention to those 'clench' traps – the toes, fingers, shoulders and jaw.
Breathe normally and, with each breath, try to slow down the inhale and the exhale.

Progressively deepen the length of each breath in and each breath out.

On each exhale, say the word 'One' to yourself (like so: W-u-n-n-n-n-n-n-n-n-n-n), either quietly or out loud. By concentrating on this single word, it helps to push intrusive thoughts away.

The 'One' sound is a good way of dealing with unwelcome 'mind chatter' and, each time you use this exercise, you should find it easier to relax.

These simple exercises can help to reduce nervous tension. Some use movement, some use the breath only. Do them regularly to help ward off stress attacks or use them as emergency measures if you are anxious at any time:

TAKE THE STRAIN FROM YOUR BRAIN

This first exercise was described and explained to me by a Chinese doctor whom I met in Singapore. It's a simple visualization exercise which helps to relax your brain. First, find a comfortable place to sit or lie down, away from noise and distractions. Make a picture in your mind of your brain and the skull bones which protect and surround it. Breathe gently but deeply. With every inhalation, imagine your brain expanding slightly so that it just touches the inside of your skull. When you exhale, picture the brain returning to its normal size. Repeat this process six times and then rest for a few minutes before resuming normal activities. This is also a useful exercise to do whilst waiting to go to sleep at night.

SIX SIMPLE EXERCISES TO HELP YOU RECHARGE YOUR BATTERIES

Try them all and then choose the ones you enjoy the most to practise regularly:

ONE: Relax in a comfortable chair. At your desk, VDU or in your car will do if you don't have an armchair to hand. With your feet placed flat on the floor and slightly apart, allow your arms to flop loosely beside you. Close your eyes, relax your jaw and your shoulders – and breathe deeply. Imagine your arms are made of lead. Let your mind wander for a few minutes. Bring yourself back to reality whenever you feel ready.

TWO: Picture yourself in a place you have enjoyed visiting: a holiday location, perhaps, a quiet garden; in fact, anywhere where you felt happy and comfortable. Alternatively, retreat to your mental refuge. Close your eyes and imagine yourself in this special place. If you can lie down or sit down, so much the better but don't worry if not. Just standing, eyes closed, breathing slowly and steadily, with the wind or the sun on your face can be unwinding in itself. Let your mind walk around your visualized setting and enjoy the sounds (bird song, a steam train, a waterfall or stream perhaps), the colours, flowers and trees, sunlight, gentle breezes or dappled shade. When you feel ready, bring yourself back to where you are by taking a deep breath and enjoy a gentle stretch and sigh.

THREE: A variation on the above visualization is to imagine that you are involved in a recreation that you enjoy; it could be cycling, swimming, sailing, surfing, skiing or just walking. Don't forget to slow and deepen your breathing. You are surrounded by beautiful blue water or wonderful countryside. You are cycling down a country lane, for example, or riding the surf or skiing your favourite slope. Feel the warmth of the sun and absorb energy from all the colours and sounds around you. When you are actually physically involved in these kinds of activities, make mental notes of sights and sounds which please you so that you can incorporate them into your visualization.

FOUR: Tension often shows in the face. Since it takes many more muscles to frown than it does to smile, it's not surprising that grimacing and glowering can increase the number of wrinkles. Always remember that cross-patch people get crow's feet but happy people get laughter lines! For this exercise, sit in the same position as above and concentrate on the face. Is your forehead frowning, are your eye muscles tight, is your jaw clamped and your teeth clenched? Let the tension go by pulling faces then relaxing, allowing the jaw to drop. Take in a deep breath, hold for a count of three and release the air in a huge sigh. With the out-breath, push away tension and anger.

FIVE: Lie down on the floor or on the bed or relax in a comfortable sitting position. Inhale deeply and sigh. Now breathe in and out through the nose. Think through your body, starting with your toes, feet, calf muscles, thigh muscles, buttocks, abdomen, chest, arms, hands, shoulders, neck, jaw, eyes and scalp. Tense each area in turn, hold for three seconds and then let go. Repeat once more. This is a good exercise to try if you have difficulty getting off to sleep.

SIX: Go for a short walk. Taking yourself away from the

area where the stress and pressure have occurred is very beneficial. Stretch and breathe as you go. Far better for your stress levels than a coffee or a chocolate bar.

BASIC BREATHING AND MOVEMENT

In these two exercises, each movement is made on either the inhalation or exhalation. Breathe slowly and deeply through the nose, without strain or force. Focus on bringing your breathing and your movement together; in other words, move in time with your breathing. There should be a very slight pause between inhaling and exhaling and, again, between exhaling and inhaling. You will find that the length of your breath may vary from day to day, depending upon your stress levels, your state of mind and your emotions. Accept this without judgement.

TAKE YOUR TIME

We all have our own individual breath length. When doing your breathing exercises, do them at your own pace. You are not taking part in a competition. What is most important is that you slow down and deepen your breathing from what it used to be, i.e. fast, shallow, tight and tense. As you progress with these exercises, try to make each exhalation a little longer than the inhalation.

Counting on the inhale and on the exhale will help you to slow the out breath. Don't count at a rapid one/two/three/four/five but at a more relaxed wunnnnn . . . , tooooo . . . , threeeee . . . , etc. If you breathe in to, say, six, then breathe out to seven and so on.

Sequence One

Photographs A1 to A6 accompany this exercise.

*** Sit on a chair which has a straight back (a dining or office chair). Choose the right height so that your thighs are almost parallel to the floor but sloping very slightly away from you. The soles of your feet should be in contact with the floor. Check that your toes are relaxed. Let your arms hang loosely beside you. Your back should be straight but not tense. *(See photo A1.)* Think about your shoulders and relax them. Begin to slow down your breathing.

*** Inhale, lifting your arms out sideways to shoulder level and with palms facing upwards. *(See photo A2.)* Pause slightly. Exhale, lowering your arms back to your starting point. Repeat six times.

*** From the same starting point *(see photo A3)*, inhale and lift your arms so that upper arms are level with the shoulders and palms are facing forwards *(see photo A4)*. Exhale, lowering the arms. Repeat six times.

*** Sit with your hands resting gently around your lower abdomen. Fingertips should be touching with palms facing inwards against your clothing. Keep the back straight but not stiff. Without putting any strain on the neck, tuck the chin gently downwards so that you can see your hands *(photo A5)*. Focus on slow, deep and steady breathing. When you breathe in and the abdomen moves forwards, feel the fingertips spread (*photo A6*). When you breathe out, see the abdomen sink and your fingertips come together again. Repeat six times and then rest.

Sequence Two

Photographs B1 to B6 accompany this exercise.

*** Lie on a rug, exercise mat or soft towel on the floor. Make sure eyelids are relaxed, not clamped shut! Place a pillow or rolled up towel under your head, neck and lower back for extra comfort if needed. With feet flat on the floor but a few inches apart, draw them towards you so that your knees are bent. Arms should be resting by your sides. (*See photograph B1.*)

*** Settle down and slow your breathing. Gradually breathe more deeply and more slowly.

*** When you are ready, inhale and lift the arms up so that they are at right angles to the body (see *photo B2*). As you move, bend the elbows a little so that there is no strain on the arms or neck. (Remember that you are not practising a salute!)

*** Exhale and lower the arms back to the starting point. Remember to keep the movement timed to your breathing. Inhale – up, exhale – down.

*** This time, inhale as before, raising the arms (*see photo B3*). When you exhale and lower the arms, bring the left knee up towards the chest (*photo B4*).

*** With arms still by your sides (*as in photo B5*), inhale again, lower the left leg and bring your foot

back to the floor. Exhale. Rest for a moment.
*** Change sides and do the same movements using the right knee. Inhale – arms up, exhale – arms down and right knee to chest. Inhale – put right foot back on the floor. Exhale. Rest. If you find this movement comfortable, repeat six times both sides.
*** For the final part of **sequence two**, remain in the same position, lying down on the floor, with knees bent and feet slightly apart. Place your hands on your lower abdomen with fingertips gently touching. *(See photo B6.)*
*** Breathe in slowly and deeply and notice the fingers moving apart as your abdomen extends.
*** Exhale as slowly as you can and feel the fingers come together again. Repeat six times.
*** Rest quietly for a few minutes.

Basic stretching exercises

••• No cheating. It is important to follow all six exercises in sequence.
••• After a few practice sessions, you'll find that, together, the whole lot will take only a couple of minutes each day.
••• Best done during the day or in the early evening. Muscles may not be so flexible first thing in the morning.
••• Don't forget that the whole point about *All Day Energy* is that it is about being yourself and giving yourself some special attention. The following exercises and simple movements are within the reach and capabilities of almost everyone – and you

won't need any special clothing, footwear or equipment.

- ••• If possible, do the movements in front of a full length mirror so that you can check your positioning.
- ••• During each stretch, check your breathing. You should be breathing naturally and normally but you may find yourself holding your breath while you are concentrating, especially during the learning period.
- ••• Fitness specialist Jan Robinson (that's Jan in the photographs with me) recommends that each stretch is held for eight seconds when you first begin. Once practised, hold for as long as you wish – *up to thirty seconds*.
- ••• Throughout the stretches, remember to B-R-E-A-T-H-E normally.
- ••• Don't ever, ever, strain. When you stretch, do it with a feeling of 'oooooh' (that's a nice stretch) but not 'owwww' (that hurts).

FIRST
Photograph C accompanies this movement.
- *** With feet parallel and hip width apart, bend the knees slightly.
- *** Link your fingers above your head, palms facing upwards.
- *** Don't worry if you can't straighten your arms fully.
- *** Push arms gently back and reach upwards.
- *** Pull in your tummy so as not to arch your back.
- *** Don't strain but feel the muscles tense in your

upper arms and shoulders and feel the sensation of 'pulling up' from the ribs and waist.
*** Hold for eight seconds.
*** Breathe naturally and normally.
*** Release and relax.

SECOND

Photograph D accompanies this movement.
*** With feet and legs in the same position as exercise 'C', bend the knees slightly as before. Link fingers again, this time in front of you, palms facing away from you and arms parallel with the floor.
*** Feel the stretch across your arms, upper back and shoulders.
*** Pull tummy in gently so as not to arch the back.
*** Hold for eight seconds.
*** Breathe naturally and normally.
*** Release and relax.

THIRD

Photograph E accompanies this movement
*** Again with feet and legs positioned as in exercises 'C' and 'D', bend the knees slightly as before.
*** Link your fingers behind your back.
*** Keep the body upright (resist the natural inclination to lean forwards or to pull the head too far back).
*** Head should stay level with chin parallel to the floor.
*** Pull shoulders back and down.
*** Tuck in your tummy, so as not to arch your back.

***   Raise the arms (with hands still linked) away from your back and lift the chest area.

Move them only a short distance.

Do not strain.

Keep elbows bent if this is more comfortable.

***   Feel the stretch across your shoulders, chest and arms.

***   Hold for eight seconds.

***   Breathe naturally and normally.

***   Release and relax.

FOURTH

Photograph F accompanies this movement.

***   With feet parallel and hip distance apart, step forward with left leg.

***   Balance yourself well.

***   Place your hands on your upper left thigh.

***   Without moving your feet again, move your body-weight slowly forward without leaning. Check your position with photograph 'F'.

***   Your right leg should be straight and your right heel pressing firmly on the ground.

***   Feel the stretch predominantly in your right calf.

***   Check your right foot; it should be facing forwards.

***   Hold for eight seconds.

***   Breathe naturally and normally.

***   Release and relax.

***   Change sides and repeat the movement, this time starting with hands resting on your right thigh

and with your left leg stretched out behind you.
*** Release and relax.

FIFTH

Photograph G accompanies this movement.
*** Do this movement deliberately and carefully.
*** Stand with feet hip width apart.
*** Step forward with your left leg. Bend your right knee.
*** In other words, the right leg should be bent, the left leg straightened in front of you with the left heel on the floor and the toes of the left foot pointing upwards.
*** Place both hands on the top of the right thigh just above the knee.
*** Lean forward a little farther and feel the stretch behind the left thigh, left knee and left calf.
*** Hold for eight seconds.
*** Breathe naturally and normally.
*** Release and relax.
*** Change sides and repeat the movement, this time starting with your hands on your left thigh and your right leg stretched out in front of you.
*** Release and relax.

SIXTH

Photograph H accompanies this movement.
*** Stand with feet parallel and hip distance apart.
*** Pull your tummy in gently so as not to arch your back, avoiding the temptation to lean forward.

***   Lift your left knee up in front of you until you can hold on to your left ankle with your left hand.

***   Do this movement slowly.
        If you cannot reach your ankle, put a soft strap around your ankle and pull on the strap instead. A sock makes a useful strap.

***   Keeping body upright, tummy in, pull on the ankle so that the left knee points towards the floor and the left heel is directed towards the left buttock.

***   Very gently and slowly, pull the heel farther towards the left buttock until you feel a good stretch in the front of the left thigh.

***   How far back you pull isn't the issue (everybody has a different level of flexibility) as long as the body is straight. In other words, check that you are not leaning forwards or arching your back. You should feel a good stretch down the front of the left thigh.

***   Don't strain.

***   Hold for eight seconds.

***   Breathe naturally and normally.

VERY IMPORTANT

If you are new to exercise, do please ask for professional assistance. If you have an existing health problem and are receiving medication, check first with your practitioner before embarking on any new fitness activity. Under any circumstances, if in doubt, ask before you begin. The exercises included in this chapter should not be attempted by anyone with a severe heart or chest condition except under medical supervision.

I'd like to reiterate my appreciation to Jan Robinson and Mary Harris for their invaluable comments and contributions to this chapter. My thanks also to The Exercise Association.

SOURCES OF REFERENCE:

~ Jain S. Effects of yoga training on exercise tolerance in adolescents with childhood asthma. *Journal of Asthma* 1991;28(6):437–42.
~ Singh V, Wisniewski A, Britton J, Tattersfield A. Effect of yoga breathing exercises (pranayama) on airway reactivity in subjects with asthma. *Lancet* 1990; 335:1381–3.
~ Caren L D. Effects of Exercise on the Human Immune System: Does Exercise Influence Susceptibility to Infections? *Bioscience* 1991;41(6):410–15.

10

Eating for Energy:
Casting off the Calorie Counting Culture

Why do so many of us spend endless amounts of time worrying about how many Calories or fat grams are in a particular food, stocking our cupboards and refrigerators with only low fat this and low cholesterol that, avoiding cream and butter, depriving ourselves of dessert and then pigging out on crisps, cakes and chocolate between meals? Could it be that, although we have a fair idea of what's good and what's not, none of us finds 'healthy food' all that inspiring or satisfying? When we're bored, stressed and tired, what solace or stamina can there be in a low fat cracker and twenty grams of cottage cheese?

If we are going to beat fatigue, we must climb down from the Calorie counting bandwagon. But it's not always easy to change the habits of a lifetime, especially if it means questioning the official, but seemingly ever changing, health dogma of the day.

WHAT IS A CALORIE, ANYWAY?

At school, most of us learn that a calorie is 'the amount of heat required to raise the temperature of one gram of water by 1°C'. 'Calorie', written with a capital 'C', actually means kilocalories or 1000 'little' calories (those with a small 'c') and so will heat a kilogram (1000 grams) of water by the same degree. You're sorry I started this, aren't you?

'Large' Calories are the units which we associate with food. The medical physiology textbooks instruct us that different types of food produce different amounts of Calorie energy. When the cells burn one gram of protein or starch (carbohydrate), four Calories of 'energy' are produced, whereas one gram of fat produces nine Calories. Physiological logic therefore dictates that, because fat has more Calories per gram than protein or starch, fat is more fattening and produces more 'energy' than protein or starch. Isn't this absolutely riveting!

So how does all that chemistry help us to understand and relate Calories to what we eat or the energy value of our food to the energy *levels* we eventually end up with? Well, it doesn't help much at all. All it really achieves is to perpetuate the myth that, somehow, Calories and fat are villains of the dietary piece.

We are particularly addicted and obsessed by Calories; confused by them; conned by them (yes, conned) and probably fed up with hearing about them but, strangely, dedicated to counting them! Now we are adding the counting of fat grams to our obsession. Almost every packeted food item we buy has the Calorie and/or kilojoule value and the number of fat grams stamped indelibly on the wrapping. Whether they are dieting or not, almost every person you know can tell you how many Calories a particular food contains; an increasing number are able to reel off the fat content; but few can quote the vitamin or mineral levels. Thanks to muddling, misleading, inconsistent labelling, no-one less than a biochemistry graduate can make sense of the ingredients.

Play a word game which begins with the word 'Calorie' and most people will connect with the word 'weight'; usually in the context of complaining about weight *gain* and wishing wistfully for weight *loss*. For them, too many Calories means too tubby; lowering Calories means lean.

Mention the word 'energy' in your word game and the majority of us will think '*LACK* of energy', bemoaning our ever-present state of fatigue. When we talk about energy in relation to food, however, the majority will link it to Calories (or kilojoules), being the measurements used to work out the 'energy' value of our food.

But how many of us link Calories *directly* to *LACK* of energy? It's the connection we would probably miss in our word game – the one which joins Calorie counting to lethargy and tiredness. If your breakfast consists of a croissant and coffee and your lunch is a low-fat yoghurt, it's no wonder you have the mental clarity of a plastic bin liner and the physical stamina of a punctured tyre. Almost everyone who has ever dieted for weight loss knows that the major handicap is an energy slump. Anybody who has gone all day without food doesn't usually have much energy left by the end of it.

ARE YOU GETTING ENOUGH?

The fact that depriving ourselves of sustenance increases the risk of being tired all the time shouldn't come as any surprise. The average adult needs between 1800 and 2200

Calories daily (depending upon age, sex, activity level, etc.) to function effectively. Go overboard on Calorie restriction and the body isn't receiving enough sustenance to supply all its needs.

How often do we consider the possibility that our number crunching dependence upon Calorie counting could also be restricting our intake of the very nutrients we need to produce energy? Whether you are reducing Calories in order to lose weight or counting them to avoid putting weight on, chances are you could be losing out on nourishment. Unless nutritional intake is very carefully monitored, dieting by Calorie restriction can be a potentially dangerous and exhausting business.

A normal, healthily balanced diet, we are advised, should be able to provide all our energy requirements. But how many of us manage to achieve that happy state? And where does that leave those who are meticulous about achieving the right intake of proteins, starches and fats, yet still suffer from unexplained lethargy and exhaustion?

BLOOD GLUCOSE BALANCE

Our actual available energy levels are related to the circulating levels of glucose in our blood. To keep those levels steady and stabilized, we need *regular* pit stops for *quality* fuel. As can be seen in the section on Hypoglycaemia, if we take in too few foods or choose the wrong kinds of Calories, circulating glucose can be affected so detrimentally that our available energy becomes very limited indeed. If you've missed breakfast or lunch and tried to survive on coffee and chocolate bars, you'll know what I mean. Next step exhaustion!

QUALITY COUNTS

It is simply not enough to judge a food by its Calorie measurement. The *quality* of those Calories, their *nutritional value*, how *efficiently* the body digests and absorbs the nourishment from them – and the speed at which they are absorbed – are all important keys to how energetic and healthy you are going to feel.

Yet, despite this knowledge, we still rely heavily on calorific value as the *only* guide to food choices, adhering strictly to the belief (albeit erroneous) which says that high Calorie foods are bad for us and low Calorie foods are good. Unfortunately, this can lead to contradiction and confusion. Not every low Calorie food is 100 per cent healthy; not every high Calorie food is bad news! Carrot Calories may be preferable to piles of cream cakes – confirmed, presumably, by the fact that Bugs Bunny has lots of stamina! But is an additive-laden, low fat, low cholesterol mayonnaise a better option than a dressing made with extra virgin olive oil? Or a low Calorie breakfast cereal which leaves you screaming with hunger by eleven a.m. more nourishing than scrambled eggs or waffles? Maybe a low Calorie, virtually fat free, stick it in the microwave, 'ready' meal really is healthier than half an avocado piled with prawns or a plate of nourishing pasta? Unlikely.

BLINKERED VIEW?

The official line is that obesity results from eating more Calories than you expend. What you don't burn off hangs on as fat. OK, there will always be people who have problems cutting down on food intake and who can't or won't exercise. But it's difficult to go along slavishly with the orthodox view that *every* overweight person is that way because they eat too much and exercise too little, the only exceptions being those with thyroid problems or other metabolic disorders linked to obesity.

I've met many overweight people who, despite unswerving dedication to Calorie controlled dieting and exercising, do not seem able to shed surplus fat. And please don't give me the line which pushes the guilt back on to the dieter; that they are eating more than they realize so it's their fault.

EVERYBODY'S DOING IT!

Dieting is an international pastime. Most people with weight problems seem to have tried most diets. Most diets revolve around Calorie values. So many people are doing it and doing it and doing it, over and over again. If calculating Calories and gauging fat grams were successful in resolving weight problems, why is the world full of people with weight problems? Obese or anorexic, the guilt, shame and failure shouldn't be loaded onto the sufferer but onto those who continually push Calorie loading or unloading as the only way to a perfect body.

EATING FOR ENERGY: FORGET THE FAT GRAMS

The furore over fat is proof positive that anyone can do anything with statistics and scientific research. First of all, saturated fat was the cause of high cholesterol. Scientific studies said so – it must be right. Change to polyunsaturated fats, give up butter and all will be well. A mere twenty years of margarine madness and an epidemic of yellow oilslicks masquerading as butter and what do we hear? Sorry, folks; we forgot to mention that the process used to make solid fat out of liquid polyunsaturated oils *may* not be so healthy after all and *may* actually increase the risk of, guess what, can you believe it? heart disease and, possibly, cancer! But it's OK to carry on eating it!?

More scientific research then takes another 180° turn – the cholesterol theory is a myth – apparently. It isn't the heart disease risk factor we once thought it was. Although saturated fat may raise cholesterol levels, the cholesterol in food has little or nothing to do with the cholesterol in our blood. But 'low in cholesterol' is still shouted from the food packaging roof tops, the inference being that anything low in cholesterol must be great news and anything high in cholesterol must be dangerous. The margarine manufacturers continue to extol the virtues of their products and a government document is issued telling us that whilst 'no evidence exists that high dietary intakes of PUFAs [polyunsaturates] have been associated with any human disease . . . the existing evidence justifies a cautious approach'. Otherwise translated as 'keeping your hedge-betting options open'. And they wonder why the consumer is confused!

Counting Calories and fat grams is such a waste of energy. Whether it's butter, lard, dripping, margarine, suet, ghee or the oil from coconut, safflower, sunflower, rapeseed, grapeseed, soya beans or olives, the Calorie values are pretty much the same. Indeed, all fat is high in Calories — but that doesn't mean we should avoid it totally. Excess amounts of saturates (the solid stuff) are likely to be deposited as extra 'static' fat, usually in some fairly undesirable places and, so, are best kept to a minimum. However, a daily intake of cold-pressed oils (rich in essential fatty acids) is vital for making membranes and hormones, for proper brain function, stress control, concentration, memory function and for guarding against mental and physical exhaustion.

SO WHAT SHOULD YOU CHOOSE AND USE?

What it comes down to, as almost always, is moderation and the avoidance not of margarine or butter but of excesses and extremes. There is plenty of evidence that eating too much fat could cause a number of different health problems but that sensible amounts of the best quality fats and oils are probably very good for us. And there's the clue: *quality*.

A great many of the cooking oils which you see on the shelves are extracted using solvents. Unfortunately, this process destroys much of the product's health benefits. Light and warmth cause further degeneration and yet most oils are displayed in a warm atmosphere in clear containers. In addition, cooking with polyunsaturated oils may damage them even further. Some researchers are concerned that oils which are heated and reheated (in a chip fryer, for example) may become potentially carcinogenic (cancer forming).

What happens to the fats or oils after you have eaten them is also important. Where the diet is low in protective anti-oxidant nutrients – such as vitamin A, vitamin C, vitamin E, selenium and zinc – fats and oils are more likely to be degraded by a process called lipid peroxidation. Once damaged, they cease to be of any nutritional value and are much more likely to clog up the arteries and increase the risk of stroke or heart attack.

But giving up fats and oils is not the answer. The oft reported instruction that everyone should cut fat intake has created its own problems. True to form, some people didn't just reduce their fat intake, they removed the stuff from their diets altogether. Now we find that lowering cholesterol too far can also be dangerous and that too little fat could lead to joint problems, exacerbated arthritis, dry skin, eczema, poor circulation and a number of other possibles – including lack of energy.

DON'T GIVE UP FAT AND OILS; YOU NEED THEM IN YOUR DIET

Use extra virgin olive oil (which is monounsaturated) for cooking, small amounts of butter for spreading and quality cold-pressed polyunsaturated oils (such as safflower, sesame or sunflower) for salad dressings. Generally, if you don't see the words 'first pressing' or 'cold pressed' on the label, then it isn't. Health food stores and delicatessens are the best places to find quality cold-pressed oils.

Steer clear of foods which have the words 'hydro-genated vegetable oils' on the label and don't go crazy over cakes, biscuits, deep-fries and take-aways. Eat plenty of fresh vegetables, salads, wholegrains, fish, seeds and nuts. That way, your fat intake should be about right and your health – and energy levels – will probably be better for it.

THIS IS WHERE IT STOPS

Forget appetite suppressants, jaw wiring and liposuction. Forget fat grams. Forget counting and weighing. And finally, forget about Calories. It's time to try a different approach.

Whether you have a 'weight problem' or not, discovering lost energy has nothing to do with Calorie counting and everything to do with enjoying your food. There is nothing more likely to sap your stamina and drag you into depression than forcing your way through a heap of allegedly good-for-you fat-free, Calorie-restricted garbage that isn't to your taste.

Scientists have established once and for all that yo-yo dieting is an extremely unhealthy activity (well, we all knew that, didn't we?). The good news is that if you are only a few pounds overweight it can be healthier to leave well alone than to strive and struggle to lose that little bit extra. Going up one size in clothes has to be a better option than gall bladder disease, heart failure or temperamental hormones which could all be on the cards if you are an habitual dieter.

EATING FOR ENERGY: HOW IS YOUR DIGESTION DOING?

Even if we shop sensibly and prepare our meals carefully, few of us would think about the food – once it has been swallowed – unless, of course, it gives us grief. Heartburn, indigestion, bloating, constipation – may all be blamed on 'something we ate' but do we pay any closer attention to our diets as a result? Hardly ever. The most usual consequence is to reach for the antacids or the laxatives. Indigestion remedies and medicines to 'make you go' might remove the immediate symptoms of discomfort but are unlikely to cure any long-term problems. Relying on them can increase the risk of vitamin and mineral deficiencies and a greater likelihood of tiredness and energy problems.

One of the major keys to improved energy and balanced bodyweight is good digestion. The reason is simple. The nutrients we need for repair and for energy are supplied by the foods we eat. If we don't digest foods properly, absorption is likely to be affected. Unfortunately for many of us, our digestive systems are under so much strain that our exhausted and over-stressed bodies are unlikely to be releasing the full value of those nutrients to the different departments in the system.

TAKE THINGS EASY

Eating on the run, bolting every mouthful, never leaving any time to relax after a meal, eating too much at one sitting: all these misdemeanours will reduce the number of nutrients absorbed. A digestive system under this amount of pressure will be drawing heavily on already limited energy reserves. In addition, the problem is likely to be exacerbated by stress, over- or under- production of stomach acid, enzyme deficiencies, lactose intolerance, leaky gut syndrome, food allergies and a number of other factors. The result of such havoc is, not surprisingly, lethargy – often coupled to a not-so-great health record.

REMEDY IN YOUR HANDS

There is plenty that can be done to help improve the digestion, reduce weariness and increase wellbeing. Read through the following list and see how many of these suggestions apply to you:

YOU DON'T CHEW YOUR FOOD PROPERLY

Ah ha! Who does? Diligent munching and crunching is where efficient digestion begins. The better use that is made of the action of teeth and saliva, the less strain will be put on the rest of your digestive system. Grandmother's advice about not loading your fork or spoon until you've chewed and swallowed what's already in the hatch is worth thinking about. A meal may take more time to consume but you are likely to gain far more from the goodies it contains if you linger longer and savour each mouthful.

YOU NEVER EAT BREAKFAST BECAUSE EITHER YOU CAN'T FACE IT OR YOU HAVEN'T LEFT ENOUGH TIME TO EAT IT

Get up a few minutes earlier in the morning and make time for breakfast. If you hate the sight or smell of food at that hour, then eat a light snack as soon as you feel able.

YOU DON'T OFTEN SIT DOWN TO MEALS – OR IF YOU DO, YOU RUSH AWAY AS SOON AS YOUR PLATE IS EMPTY

Guilty as charged! Women are often the worst offenders, too; feeling pressured to get back to the office, the washing up, the next course, the searching for whatever it is the master/boss/partner/child can't locate. A tense stomach is unlikely to be able to cope as well with a meal than one which is relaxed. It really is worth taking the time to stop for food and take a proper break. Sit for ten minutes when you've finished eating and don't take vigorous exercise immediately after food. If you eat in a family group, don't always feel pressured to get up from the table to attend to someone else's demands. You're not a slave.

YOU'RE ALWAYS WOUND UP TO FEVER PITCH

Not great news for the digestion either as it can cause imbalances in the production of stomach acid. From the symptoms they describe, many stressed individuals seem to produce too much stomach acid between meals (when it isn't needed) and too little when it *is* required, when they eat. Slow down, take a few deep breaths before you settle into your victuals and, if at all possible, put work out of your mind for the duration of the meal. If, however, your life is one round of working breakfasts, business lunches or restaurant dinners, try to avoid rich sauces and deep fried food. Select extra vegetables or salads and light desserts. Don't allow yourself to be rushed.

YOU GALLOP FROM ONE COURSE TO ANOTHER WITHOUT PAUSING FOR BREATH

Another little tip which helps to take the strain off the system is to allow five or ten minutes between courses. If there really isn't much time to do this, then eat one course only and save any others for later, or eat 'little but more often'.

YOU DON'T HAVE TIME TO EAT DURING THE DAY SO YOU MAKE UP FOR IT BY HAVING A LARGE MEAL IN THE EVENING

Studies show that eating little and often is healthier for several reasons. Blood glucose balance is maintained; energy levels are generally higher; smaller, more frequent meals help to keep cholesterol in check. Grazing is also said to be better for weight control than gorging! In addition, large meals divert blood away from the brain to the stomach, leaving you feeling slow and slothful. And mega meals late at night are unlikely to be properly digested, increasing the risk of poor quality sleep. It's up to you!

YOU OFTEN EAT A PIECE OF FRUIT OR A FRUIT SALAD FOR DESSERT BECAUSE YOU BELIEVE IT'S A HEALTHY THING TO DO

Yes and no. Fruit is packed with nourishment but if you push it down the tubes too soon after the main course, you could cause indigestion and bloating. The reason is that fruit likes to pass quickly through the stomach but, if baulked by the more slowly-digested proteins or starches, it can ferment and cause distension, pain and flatulence. Fruit can also delay the digestion of other foods. It's good to eat plenty of fresh fruit but best to treat it as either a starter to a meal or a between meal snack – or as a mixed fruit platter on its own. Otherwise, delay the fruit dessert for an hour after the main course. If you enjoy fruit juices, drink them before meals, not with and not immediately afterwards.

YOU'RE TOO BUSY LOOKING AFTER OTHER PEOPLE TO WORRY ABOUT YOUR OWN MEALS. CONSEQUENTLY, YOU USUALLY END UP WITH LEFTOVERS AND LIMITED CHOICES

You owe it to yourself to eat as wide a variety of foods as possible. Sticking to only a few of the same old faithfuls may seem a short cut when you're pushed for time but restricted choices can result in too few nutrients. Cutting back on variety may also increase the risk of food intolerance. Redress the balance by promising yourself a new introduction to your existing menu each week. Be a bit more adventurous and try something you haven't tried before. The supermarkets and grocery stores are full of good ideas.

YOU ALWAYS DRINK LOTS OF FLUID AT MEALTIMES

For some people, large quantities of liquid with food can cause indigestion and bloating. If this applies to you, try drinking before you eat — or waiting for 30 to 60 minutes after food before you drink. A glass of wine or water with a meal is usually beneficial; it's the larger amounts which seem to cause digestive disturbance.

YOU SEEM TO DRINK TEA AND COFFEE ALMOST EVERY HOUR OF THE DAY

There would appear to be about as many studies extolling the benefits of tea and coffee as there are telling us about their detrimental effects. In moderate amounts, these kinds of beverages can be enjoyable, even beneficial. One cup of coffee can perk you up for as long as two hours. A cup of tea can be the treat which gets you through the afternoon. On the hour every hour, however, caffeine-laden drinks can encourage nutritional deficiencies and will probably leave you feeling wiped out. Why not take the opportunity to swap a few teas and coffees for more water and fresh juices?

YOU OFTEN SUFFER FROM SERIOUS PANGS OF HUNGER DURING THE DAY

If you feel hungry and the next mealtime is way off, then you could be doing more harm than good by denying yourself some food. Stomach pain or heartburn are common symptoms in such circumstances; a drop in energy levels is almost inevitable. A light snack or drink may be all that is needed to restore comfort.

YOU FEEL LIKE A BLOATED BAG OF WIND

Gas, flatulence, IBS, constipation and diarrhoea are common problems? First of all, put the other tips in this chapter into practice and see if the situation improves. Chewing food properly, improving your diet, avoiding sugar, yeast, cow's milk and wheat products, separating proteins from starches (next section), eating fruit between – not with – meals and taking a course of acidophilus supplements (page 355) should all be priorities. You'll find information on each of these points throughout *All Day Energy*. If there is no improvement after four to six weeks, then see your doctor for a check-up and ask to be referred to a practitioner who is familiar with the treatment of candidiasis and intestinal (gut) dysbiosis. See How to Find a Practitioner on page 352.

FOOD COMBINING FOR ENERGY

Surprising as it may seem, how we combine our food at each mealtime really can affect our energy levels – because it improves the way we digest and absorb nourishment.

The first time that I tried Food Combining was in the early 1980s when my husband was desperately ill and fighting for his life. Since then, I have seen this enjoyable, common-sense way of eating help not just Ralph but many, many other people too. Some were faced with chronic illness, others had endured apparently intractable weight problems, countless numbers were suffering from fatigue, exhaustion and stress. What they have in common, however, is that they give Food Combining the major credit for their restored health. Those suffering the pain and discomfort associated with digestive and bowel disorders seem particularly improved.

Sometimes, short-term Food Combining is all that is needed to put someone on the road to recovery. Other times, longer term care is required. Diet is not a cure-all and there is no system that will be 100 per cent effective for everybody. However, for a great many people, Food Combining has become, quite literally, a way of life. These are two typical responses:

••• For many years, I suffered bouts of indifferent health, stress and nervous tension and never felt full of beans. I saw your book [*The Food Combining Diet*] advertised so feeling I had nothing left to lose I started in a small way, separating proteins and starches and eating lots more fruit, vegetables and salad. I can say I now feel heaps better (I lost seven pounds in the first two weeks) and intend to carry on with the good work. I find the menus easy to follow and there are no complicated foods to purchase.

••• I listened with interest to your contribution to the BBC Radio 4 *Food Programme*. Despite several allergies and food intolerances, I adopted the food combining

274

approach. My weight loss was slow but steady and I am pleased to have lost nearly all 'repeating' and indigestion. Also, I no longer suffer from travel sickness. I am sure you are 100 per cent right to advocate alteration to diet as a preventive measure — so much better than taking medicines.

For reasons best known to themselves, a mini-clique of conventionally trained medics and dietitians seem to enjoy decrying Food Combining. A minority have made such a 'career' out of knocking its benefits that I have to wonder when they find time to get any real work done. There are none so blind as those who *can* see, but won't, runs the old proverb!

I have quoted, before, the perceptive words of Dr Walter Yellowlees, who reminds us that academic specialists are not always wise counsellors. They may distort evidence in order to further their own particular theory and tend to escape contentious issues by falling back on the verdict Not Proven.

The proof of Food Combining is in the results and, over the years, it has received much acclaim; in a great number of cases, working where no other treatments have been effective.

WHY THE MIX MATTERS

Protein foods will not be broken down without stomach acid. On the other hand, carbohydrates (starches) need an alkaline environment, preferring the stomach to remain non-acidic for the first stages of digestion. Mix the two together and, food combiners believe and chemistry students will confirm, the acids and alkalis cancel each other out. Result: considerably curtailed digestion.

Most experts agree that the miracle of human digestion is a very long way from being completely understood. When something goes wrong, the most usual treatments will be drug medication or surgery. Dietary advice, if it is given at all, is still way down the list of considerations. And yet improved eating habits have helped many people manage their condition without medicines or operations.

SIMPLICITY ITSELF

Food Combining has been written about by many different practitioners and authors. My particular style of Food Combining was introduced to simplify the system and to take account of the fact that the vast majority of us just don't have the time or inclination to cope with complicated rules or intricate recipes. My husband admits that he would never have found the resolve to stick to anything but the most straightforward of menus, yet he manages Food Combining with ease and says that if he can follow it, anybody can!

If you decide to give Kathryn Marsden's Food Combining a try, introduce it into your normal routine for just one or two days a week. Once you are familiar with the basics, you might decide to increase this to three, four or five days. Don't put yourself under any undue pressure. Healthy eating should not be treated as a cult religion! 'Indulgence days' are actively encouraged!

HERE'S WHAT TO DO:

***   AVOID MIXING *CONCENTRATED* PRO-
TEINS AND *CONCENTRATED* STARCHES
AT THE SAME MEAL
(Use the food suggestions in pages 279 and
284–292 as a guide)

***   INCREASE YOUR INTAKE OF FRESH FRUIT.
ENJOY IT EITHER BETWEEN MEALS OR AS
A STARTER – NOT WITH YOUR PROTEINS
OR STARCHES

***   DRINK PLENTY OF WATER BETWEEN
MEALS

***   DO WHATEVER YOU CAN TO CUT DOWN
ON THE ENERGY-SAPPING FOODS LISTED
ON PAGES 284–285

***   As a natural consequence of Food Combining,
you'll find that you automatically eat more vegetable and salad foods and, at the same time, eat
less packaged and processed food.

EVERY DAY, AIM FOR:

***   *One protein-based meal served with plenty of fresh veg-
etables or salad*

***   *One starch-based meal served with a good-sized portion
of fresh vegetables or salad*

and

***   *One meal based on any of the vegetable dishes which begin
on page 287 or on a selection of any fresh fruits*

This three-meal combination seems particularly helpful to those with weight problems.

Remember that the more slowly you lose weight, the less likely it is to creep back, especially if you exercise regularly and food combine several days each week.

If you don't need to shed any extra pounds, try the alternative of:

*** One protein-based meal and two starch-based meals per day accompanied by generous portions of salad or vegetables.

*** If you are hungry between meals, then it's good to snack on fresh fruit or a handful of dried fruit, nuts or seeds.

QUICK REFERENCE CHART FOR FOOD COMBINERS

Proteins in **Column A** will mix with anything from **Column B**

Starches in **Column C** will mix with anything from **Column B** but don't mix **Column A** with **Column C**.

COLUMN A PROTEINS	COLUMN B MIX WITH ANYTHING	COLUMN C STARCHES
Fish	All vegetables — except the starchy ones in Column C	Potatoes and sweet potatoes
Shellfish	All salads	All grains including: oats, pasta, brown rice, rye, millet, couscous, quinoa, bulgur
Free-range eggs	Seeds	
Free-range poultry	Nuts	
Lean lamb	Herbs	Sweetcorn
Rabbit	Fats & Oils including: cream, butter, margarine and extra virgin olive oil	Flour
Cheese		Bread & crackers
Yoghurt		Pastry
Soya beans & all soya products		
Milk — keep to a minimum and use in beverages only		

Pulses (other than soya) are an excellent source of nourishment and should be included regularly in the diet. They combine well with all kinds of vegetables and salads — and with starches — but can cause digestive problems if mixed with protein foods.

EATING FOR ENERGY: AVOIDING FOOD FATIGUE

There are a few foods that display a nasty tendency to make some of us even more tired and lethargic. Any food which is slow to digest or that the body has difficulty dealing with is likely to 'steal' energy as it works its way through your tubes. If you are already struggling for energy, the wrong diet can definitely add to your exhaustion.

If you are really interested in improving energy levels, try to cut down on the items listed on page 284. They're not called energy sappers for nothing and are included for good reason. Some cause allergic reactions, others are mucus-forming, many are high in not-so-healthy fats or sugars or have been associated directly or indirectly with one or more health problems. Some are high in Calories, others are not so high. Proving again that the Calorie value has little or no bearing on ultimate vitality.

There's no need to give them up completely, just moderate your intake and see if your energy levels improve. If a tired patch hits you, it can be an interesting (and revealing!) exercise to note the foods which you have eaten in the previous forty-eight hours and see if a pattern emerges! And don't dismiss the possibility out of hand — the food/fatigue connection may not immediately be obvious but is an increasingly common problem.

STAFF OF LIFE OR SLEEP-INDUCING LOAF?

Bread is a good example of this interesting phenomenon.

Generally regarded as the staff of life, bread – and a variety of other wheat-based products such as breakfast cereals, biscuits and cakes – form a major part of many a daily menu. The UK Health of the Nation initiative encourages us to increase our consumption of bread, believing it to be one of the best sources of starch and dietary fibre. That may be so.

Or maybe not. Unfortunately, some wheat products – especially the very 'squashy' loaves which are short on flavour but high on fresh air – can be difficult to digest and nothing less than soporific. Made using rapid fermentation methods (the bread rises in minutes instead of hours) and containing three of the most common allergens – bread wheat, yeast and gluten – the ingredients are geared to mass production using constituents that are very different from early wild wheat grains. For many people, the worst thing since sliced bread is 'bread fatigue'. But how many of us would think to connect the lethargy and sleepiness which so often follows the breakfast toast or the lunchtime sandwiches with the bread we used to make them?

I fell across this discovery quite by accident several years ago. One particular patient, when completing the section in my health questionnaire which asks 'Are there any foods which appear to upset or disagree with you?', replied 'No, but bread makes me sleepy, so I eat rice cakes instead.'

Eureka! Pennies plummeted fortissimo in my breadbefuddled brain. Was my faithful lunchtime sandwich, languishing somewhere in my digestive system like a lump of cement, one of the things dragging me into the arms of Morpheus in the middle of the afternoon? I changed to rice cakes, rye crackers and pumpernickel and my sleepiness definitely diminished. Proving that practitioners often learn more from their patients than they do from their tutors.

'Rice cakes' you say? Isn't that a bit like eating polystyrene ceiling tiles? Well, that's what rice cakes look like. But with tasty toppings, they can be very good indeed. Other delicious alternatives are yeast-free soda breads, wholemeal pitta, sourdough loaves, pasta and old-fashioned wheat grains such as spelt. If you are unsure, a general rule to follow is 'the closer the texture the better the bread'. If it's springy enough to use as a cushion, then it's probably best avoided by anyone with an iffy digestion, an energy problem, a bowel disorder or suspected food intolerances. Those who find they cannot tolerate any kind of wheat could try pumpernickel, light rye, oatcakes, rye crackers, porridge and oat-based muesli. Couscous, kamut, quinoa, millet, oats, barley and brown rice are also useful alternatives. For those who don't have a local source of any of these more unusual foods, page 349 has details of mail order suppliers.

A SLUGGISH BOWEL CAN SAP YOUR STAMINA

Dare I whisper the words *constipation* and *irritable bowel syndrome* just once more? As we've already mentioned, if efficiency isn't what it could be in that department, then tiredness, listlessness and lethargy are likely consequences. But did you know that, despite being recommended as a useful laxative, wheat fibre can make matters far worse. A daily tablespoon of linseeds with a glass of water is an excellent (and very healthy) substitute for the loathsome wheat bran sawdust and will 'get you going' gently and efficiently!

FAT AND FATIGUE

Diets which are too high in saturated fat can increase mental and physical fatigue and may also affect mood. That's why cutting down on the solid fats and increasing the cold-pressed oils in your diet can be helpful if tiredness and depression are affecting you.

That reminds me of the olive oil story. For those of you who have not been privy to my husband's birth certificate, he was (once upon a time when the Beatles were babies) a 'dyed-in-the-wool', meat-and-two-veg, chip-butties rule OK, fry everything in lard, vegetables are green things which animals eat, Liverpool man.

During the period of our own personal dietary change, I decided it was best to avoid any public declaration that I was changing lard for olive oil for fear of bringing on a relapse in my convalescing Scouse* spouse.

So, surreptitiously, I chucked out the chip pan, purchased quantities of green/gold extra virgin olive oil and sautéed the sliced potatoes (with the skins still on) in the

---

* Scouse is a colloquial expression meaning a native of Liverpool, a crazy city in the north-west of England which produces so many of our great comedians. Chip butties are an essentially northern British speciality of large sticks of deep fried potato in slices of white bread: a chip sandwich. Now generally considered to be unhealthy, fattening and bad for the heart but still one of the most delicious meals known to man/woman.

oil instead of the lard. Compliments all round and a general consensus that the chips taste really great lately! One day, Ralph ventured into the kitchen, caught me pouring olive oil into a pan and asked me why I was cooking with brake fluid. I admitted my deception and explained that I'd been using olive oil for almost a year, not just for sauté potatoes but for all kinds of other foods too. The protests faded and, surprise, surprise, he has become a great fan of olive oil.

Motto: Never judge a book by its cover or a new food only by its appearance!

CUT DOWN ON THESE ENERGY-SAPPING FOODS

SWEETS, CHOCOLATE, SUGAR AND
  SUGARY FOODS

ARTIFICIAL SWEETENERS AND FOOD OR
  DRINK WHICH CONTAINS THEM

ARTIFICIAL COLOURS, FLAVOURS AND
  PRESERVATIVES

REFINED WHITE FLOUR AND FOODS
  MADE FROM IT

TOO MUCH CAFFEINE – COFFEE, TEA,
  COCOA, COLA, HOT CHOCOLATE

ALCOHOL – ENJOY GOOD WINE IN
  MODERATION BUT GO EASY ON BEER,
  LAGER AND SPIRITS

ORANGE JUICE

PEANUTS

COW'S MILK

SOYA MILK
SOME TYPES OF BREAD – see above
WHEAT-BASED BREAKFAST CEREALS –
   check the labels
SUGAR-LOADED BREAKFAST CEREALS –
   ditto
ANYTHING DEEP FRIED
CHARCOALED, BURNED FOODS OR
   SMOKED FOODS
POLYUNSATURATED SPREADS
COOKING OILS WHICH ARE NOT COLD-
   PRESSED (check the label)
DIET FOODS
SALT AND SALTY FOODS
PORK, BEEF AND PRODUCTS WHICH
   INCLUDE THEM
BATTERY- OR BARN-RAISED POULTRY
BATTERY AND BARN EGGS
PROCESSED, SMOKED, COLOURED
   CHEESES
LOW FAT CHEESES, SPREADS,
   MAYONNAISES, ETC. WHICH CONTAIN
   ADDITIVES
See below for the healthier alternatives

EATING FOR ENERGY: THE HEALTHIER ALTERNATIVES

In this Eating for Energy section of *All Day Energy* you'll find a feast of food choices which, if used in conjunction with the other lifestyle features in the book, should help increase your energy and keep your weight in balance. For those interested in food combining (see page 273), the 'healthy alternatives' given here are divided into concentrated proteins and concentrated starches. But if you are not interested in separating proteins from starches, then that's fine too.

GOOD FOR YOU – PROTEINS

BUTTERMILK
CANNED SALMON
CANNED SARDINES
CHEESE
FREE-RANGE EGGS
FREE-RANGE POULTRY
FRESH FISH
LAMB'S LIVER
LEAN LAMB
SHELLFISH
SOYA BEANS
TOFU/BEAN CURD
YOGHURT

GOOD FOR YOU – STARCHES

BARLEY
BROWN RICE
BULGUR WHEAT
COUSCOUS

JACKET POTATOES
KASHA (Buckwheat groats)
MILLET
OATS
OAT-BASED CEREALS
OAT MUESLI
OAT PORRIDGE
PASTA
QUINOA
RICE CAKES
RYE BREAD/PUMPERNICKEL
RYE CRACKERS
SAUTÉ POTATOES
SWEET POTATOES

GOOD FOR YOU – VERSATILE VEGETABLES

The Salad, Stir-fry, Soup and Compôte which follow can be prepared in an almost infinite number of variations. Add them to any main meal or use them on their own as sustaining snacks.

There is no restriction on portion sizes. Prepare sufficient food so that, at the end of your meal, you feel comfortably sustained, not bloated and overloaded.

The foods are inexpensive, quick to prepare and full of nourishment and energy. If there is an item not to your taste, then leave it out and add another instead.

The soup and the salad travel well if stored in suitable containers – making useful alternatives to the ubiquitous and often boring sandwich.

A few examples:

Versatile salad	+	hot or cold pasta
Versatile salad	+	cheese
Versatile stir-fry	+	prawns
Versatile soup	+	rye or pitta bread
Versatile vegetable compôte	+	brown rice
Versatile salad	+	grilled fish
Versatile stir-fry	+	sauté breast of chicken
Versatile vegetable compôte	+	lamb chops
Versatile soup		followed by jacket potato
Vegetable compôte or Vegetable stir-fry		served with jacket potato

VERSATILE SALAD

Make a mixed salad using any of the following ingredients. Items should be grated, chopped or sliced as appropriate. Use your favourite dressing or leave plain.

Avocado

Beetroot (preferably raw or home-cooked, not pre packaged)

Broccoli florets

White cabbage

Carrot

Cauliflower florets

Celery

Chicory

Chinese leaves

Courgette
Skinned cucumber
Dandelion leaves
Any dark-leaved lettuce
Green, red or yellow peppers (capsicums)
Radish
Rocket
Young spinach leaves
Spring onions
Sprouted seeds
Skinned tomatoes
Watercress
Any fresh culinary herbs

VERSATILE VEGETABLE SOUP

Choose at least four items from the following list and chop
into chunks. Put them in a large pan and cover with filtered water. Bring to the boil and then simmer until
tender. Allow to cool a little (until it's safe to liquidize).
Then put the contents of the pan, including the liquid,
into a blender.

If you like a 'chunky' soup, blend only for a short time.
If a smooth soup is your fancy, leave the motor running for
longer. Return to the pan and heat through thoroughly.

Just before serving, stir in a dessertspoon of extra virgin olive oil, a dash of soy sauce, black pepper and sea salt
to taste.

Artichoke (Jerusalem)
Carrot
Courgette

Leek
Onion
Parnsip
Swede
Turnip
(Add a clove of freshly crushed garlic to the cooking – if you like garlic!)

VERSATILE STIR-FRY

Choose as many ingredients as possible:
   One tablespoon extra virgin olive oil
   Clove of crushed garlic
   A small amount of finely grated ginger
   Grated carrot
   Finely sliced celery
   Broccoli florets (break them up into very small pieces)
   Finely sliced green, red or yellow peppers (capsicums)
   Finely sliced spring onions
   Mange-tout (snow peas)
   Grated courgette
   Any sprouted seeds
   Chopped young spinach leaves
   A shake of soy sauce
   Black pepper and sea salt to taste
   Optional:
      Three teaspoons of pumpkin seeds
      Three teaspoons of sunflower seeds

Heat the olive oil in a wok or pan. Fry the garlic and the ginger for one minute. Add the carrot, celery, broccoli, peppers, spring onions, mangetout and courgette.

Cook for a further three to four minutes. Add the sprouted seeds, spinach leaves and seasoning. Turn a few times so that all the ingredients are mixed. Serve immediately.

If you like a bit more 'crunch' in your stir-fry, add the pumpkin and sunflower seeds just before serving.

VERSATILE VEGETABLE COMPÔTE

You will need evenly-sized pieces of
    Broccoli florets (and stalks if they are young and
        tender)
    Carrot
    Cauliflower florets (as for broccoli)
    Celery
    Courgette
    Kohlrabi
    Leek
    Onion

Place all ingredients into a steamer (or use a pan with a tight fitting lid so that you have only to add the minimum amount of water) and cook the compôte until just tender.

Serve on its own with a little butter or a dressing made from extra virgin olive oil and cider vinegar.

Or sprinkle with grated cheese for a tasty and filling snack.

Or serve as a main course with pasta, couscous, brown rice or jacket potato; or with lamb casserole or any kind of bean bake.

For a **Versatile Vegetable Casserole**, use the same ingredients as for the Vegetable Compôte. Add vegetable stock and cook in an oven casserole until tender.

SOURCES OF REFERENCE:

Orange Juice Fraud. Article in *The Food Magazine* April/June 1991:15, The Food Commission.

The Salt Sellers. Article in *The Food Magazine* July/Sept 1991:14–15, The Food Commission.

Can diet products help you slim? Article in *The Food Magazine* July/Sept 1991:17, The Food Commission.

The Slimming Scandal. Article in *The Food Magazine* Feb/April 1992:8–9. The Food Commission.

Roberts H J. Reactions attributed to aspartame-containing products: 551 cases. *Journal of Applied Nutrition* 1988;40:45–94.

Campion K. Dial M for Milk. Article in *What Doctors Don't Tell You* 1994;5(1):12.

Collins A M et al. Bovine milk, including pasteurized milk, contains antibodies directed against allergens of clinical importance to man. *International Archives of Allergy & Applied Immunology* 1991;96:362–7.

Ziegler E E, Fomon S J, Nelson S E, Rebouche C J, Edwards B B et al. Cow's milk feeding in infancy; further observations on blood loss from gastrointestinal tract. *Journal of Pediatrics* 1990;116:11–18.

Fernandes C F, Shahani K M. Lactose intolerance and its modulation with lactobacilli and other microbial supplements. *Journal of Applied Nutrition* 1989;41(2):50–61.

Costello J. Milk and sugar – the first drugs. *Townsend*

Letter for Doctors December 1991,1050.

Jukka Karjalainen et al. A Bovine Albumin Peptide as a Possible Trigger of Insulin-Dependent Diabetes Mellitus. *New England Journal of Medicine* 1992;327:302–97.

Sheikh M S et al. Gastrointestinal absorption of calcium from milk and calcium salts. *Journal of Nutrition* 1972;317:532–6.

Dietary Reference Values for Food Energy and Nutrients for the United Kingdom. Report of the Panel on Dietary Reference Values of the Committee on Medical Aspects of Food Policy. Department of Health Report on Health and Social Subjects 41, HMSO 1991.

Fifth International Colloquium on Monounsaturated Fatty Acids. 17 & 18 February 1992.

Willett W C, Stampfer M J, Manson J E, Colditz G A, Speizer F E, Rosner B A, Sampson L A, Hennekens C H. Intake of *trans* fatty acids and risk of coronary heart disease among women. *Lancet* 1993;341:581–5.

Smith Bob L. Organic Foods vs Supermarket Foods: Element Levels. *Journal of Applied Nutrition* 1993;45(1):35–9.

Food and Healing by A. Colbine, Ballantine Books (pp.148–60).

Free Radicals and Food Additives by B. Halliwell, Taylor & Francis, 1991.

The Composition of Foods edited by McCance and Widdowson, Fifth edition, Royal Society of Chemistry, 1992.

Food Combining in 30 Days by Kathryn Marsden. Thorsons, 1994 (pp.106–16).

The Dictionary of Vitamins by L. Mervyn, Thorsons, 1984.

The Dictionary of Minerals by L. Mervyn, Thorsons, 1985.

11

Tired and Toxic?

'Nothing can afford us more gustatory happiness and real deep-down taste contentment than a meal of luscious fruits. Such a meal is always an invitation to pleasure. A fruit meal will not cause the troubles that flow from eating fruits with other foods. Such a meal will not demoralize digestion. It will do most for you. It is both refreshing and nourishing.'

Dr Herbert Shelton,
Food Combining expert and author of Food Combining Made Easy.

Another of the many reasons for sluggishness, lethargy and general lack of energy can be toxicity. Although the very word 'toxic' conjures powerful pictures of nuclear fallout, chemical spillage, stagnant sewage and polluted rivers, it can also apply to the internal workings of the body. Your body accumulates lots of undesirable debris from a variety of different – and probably unavoidable – sources.

For example, how many people manage to escape the build-up of prescription drug residues, cigarette smoke, air pollution, too much salt and sugar, food additives and pesticides as well as internal metabolic wastes? Add other stressors such as lack of sleep, overwork, overeating, al-cohol, cigarettes, snacking on junk, wasted worry and negative thinking and your system is likely to be stretched to the limit. You could be overdue for an over-haul! But take it easy. *This is no time to launch into a potentially stressful, difficult to follow dieting nightmare.* In addition to a good diet, occasional use of liver cleansing (and immune boosting) herbs can be a positive health benefit. More information follows in the next chapter. (See also Supplement suppliers, page 355).

The trick is to enjoy the experience, to detox sensibly and avoid extremes. A well-planned spring clean has obvious and visible benefits. It's a wonderful way to reduce bloating and fluid retention, to lose a few pounds, to give your skin a glow and to bring back that lost vitality.

There are hidden plus points too. Detoxing allows every organ, gland, tissue and cell the chance to relax, unwind, repair and recharge. It's also a healthy route to resting your overworked liver and digestive system, improving bowel function (nothing like a detox to stimulate the seriously constipated!) and strengthening your immunity. Did you know that one of the best ways of dealing with a cold virus is twenty-four hours of cleansing fruits, vegetable soups and juices?

HOW LONG SHOULD THE CLEAN-UP LAST?

Forget the old adage that you have to suffer to be beautiful. Realistic and effective detoxification has nothing to do with lying on a bed of nails for days at a time, taking water only or dying between meals. My experience is that regular short detox sessions are far more convenient, easier (and fun) to do and can be more beneficial in the long run. They may also encourage you to eat more healthily the rest of the time!

GIVE YOUR BODY A BREAK

During the week before your first two cleansing days, make every effort to cut down on tea, coffee, cola and other canned fizz, alcohol, salt, sugar, sugary foods, pork, beef, yeast, wheat-based products and cow's milk. All these items can put additional strain on the body – especially the digestive and endocrine systems – and are best kept to a minimum in any healthy eating programme but especially during detoxing.

WHEN TO DETOX

The best way to begin is to choose a couple of days when you are under less pressure or don't have quite so much to do. Repeat the process approximately a week later. Then introduce a regular two-day clean-up every month or so throughout the year.

Detoxing is a terrific way to trigger weight loss, especially if you are stuck with the stuff that sticks! Some practitioners are convinced that toxicity can be a major handicap to successful dieting. But remember that the more slowly the pounds come off, the less likely they are to creep back! That's why short but regular detox sessions can be healthier – and easier on your metabolic rate – than stints of a week or a month at a time.

YOUR PRIVATE TIME

Don't use your detox days as an excuse to catch up on the

housework. Remember that this is private time – for you to look after yourself. Rest and relax as much as possible. If the weather permits, take a short walk and get some fresh air. And sleep with the window open unless you live right on the edge of a busy road.

TAKE CARE WHEN EXERCISING

Heavy aerobic sessions are not recommended during detoxing but gentle stretching exercises (see pages 249–255) can be particularly beneficial to a cleansing diet, helping to tone the system and improve circulation, carry more nutrients to the tissues and remove waste products for elimination.

WHAT TO EAT AND WHAT NOT?

For the duration, avoid heavy proteins (such as meat, milk, fish and eggs), all heavy starches (i.e. bread, pasta, cereals) and any kind of fatty or fried food. To digest these foods, your body uses lots of energy.

Focus on the foods which are easier to digest and which help most to neutralize toxins and speed elimination: fresh fruits, fresh vegetables and salads, water, juices, extra virgin olive oil, brown rice and live yogurt are the goodies which, in my experience, are the most useful.

Forget about normal mealtimes. Eat when you are hungry and drink when you are thirsty, choosing your foods and beverages from the suggestions on pages 299–304. The whole point about these two days is that the foods should be simple to prepare, flexible and satisfying. Adapt the recommendations to suit yourself.

IMPORTANT HEALTH NOTE

If you do experience a mild headache, loose bowel or slight nausea, this is a likely sign that the cleansing process is working. If symptoms persist for more than twenty-four hours, stop the detox and try again a few days later when you feel better. Taking painkillers or antacids may remove the symptoms but will give toxins the excuse they need to go back into the tissues, thereby reversing the beneficial elimination process.

This programme is not suitable for diabetics or anyone with kidney disease unless they are being medically supervised. Don't detox if you are pregnant, have an eating disorder such as anorexia or bulimia or are recovering from alcohol or drug dependency.

CLEANSING BREAKFASTS
A large fresh fruit compôte. You'll need more than one piece of fruit for this meal. Choose any combination. Eat until you are comfortably full.
Or a large glass of home-juiced fruit. See page 302.

SNACK TIME ANYTIME
A good handful of unblanched almonds, Brazil nuts, walnuts, cashews, macadamia nuts, pecans, sunflower seeds, pumpkin seeds, a few dried figs or any kind of fresh fruit. A cup of herbal tea or glass of water.

FOR MAIN COURSES
Large portion of steamed vegetables
Large bowl of home-made vegetable soup
Vegetable stir-fry (cooked in olive oil)
Steamed or gently boiled vegetables
or
A huge salad
Ideas on pages 301–302.

FOR LIGHT MEALS
A whole avocado with a tablespoon of hummus and
    sliced skinned cucumber
Organic potato baked in its jacket, dressed with
    extra virgin olive oil and cider vinegar
Crudités with yoghurt or curd cheese dip
Home-made vegetable soup
or
Any salad foods.
Add a good-sized portion of brown rice to either your
lunch or dinner.

BEFORE BED
Small carton of fresh plain (full fat) live yoghurt made
from sheep's or goat's milk. Best on its own or can be
sweetened with a teaspoon of cold-pressed New Zealand
Manuka honey (available from health food stores).

Any fruits, vegetables or salad foods are allowed during
your cleansing days. Here are just a few suggestions:

FRUIT IDEAS
Apples, fresh apricots, soaked Hunza apricots (most

health food stores have them), bananas, blackberries, blueberries, cantaloup melon, cherries, dates, figs, grapefruit, grapes, guava, honeydew melon, kiwi fruit, mangoes, nectarines, papaya, peaches, pears, pineapple, plums, pomegranates, raspberries, watermelon.

FOR SOUPS, STIR-FRYS OR FOR STEAMING
Globe artichokes, asparagus, bamboo shoots, broccoli, Brussels sprouts, cabbage, calabrese, carrots, cauliflower, cauliflower greens, celeriac, celery, leeks, marrow, pumpkin, onions, swede, turnips, turnip greens. Beans and lentils make nourishing and filling additions to winter soups.

SALAD IDEAS
Sliced apple, avocado, raw beetroot, broccoli florets, grated cabbage, grated carrot, cauliflower florets, celery, chicory, Chinese leaves, courgette, cucumber, any kind of dark leaved lettuce, bell peppers (capsicums), rocket, walnuts or watercress, fenugreek seeds, sunflower or pumpkin seeds, any fresh herbs. If you like raw onion or garlic, add those too. For dressing, avoid mayonnaise and use extra virgin olive oil with either organic cider vinegar or fresh lemon juice. Salads are generally tastier if ingredients are finely sliced or chopped and tomatoes and cucumber skinned.

TRY THESE TASTY MIXES

Grated carrot and apple with chopped celery and walnuts. Sunflower seeds with watercress, rocket, grated cabbage, chopped cucumber and pine nuts.

Half an avocado filled with hummus and topped with skinned cucumber slices.

Apple slices with dried figs and walnuts.

Skinned, sliced tomatoes with chopped basil, parsley and safflower oil.

Grated apple, raw beetroot, carrot and watercress.

Sticks of carrot and tiny florets of broccoli and cauliflower dipped in hummus.

Sliced avocado and skinned tomato with chopped bell peppers.

EXTRA REMINDERS

***   Wash all fruit and vegetables thoroughly before use. If you think something might be waxed or sprayed, then peel it too.

***   Don't go in for fasting (water only) unless you have plenty of experience or are being medically supervised.

JUICING

Properly prepared juices are not only cleansing but tasty, filling, easy to make and packed with natural enzymes, vitamins and minerals. The cartoned and bottled stuff may seem like a healthy short cut. Unfortunately, however, some brands are very acidic and may contain less fruit than you think. A few will also be well-endowed with sweeteners and colourings.

Juicing at home is a brilliant alternative. Once you've done it, you'll be hooked. Most fresh fruits make great juice drinks and, if you invest in the right juicing machine, you can make vegetable juices too. A fresh juice makes a great start to the day or a tasty aperitif while you are preparing the dinner in the evening. And they're terrific remedies for hangovers, too!

For best absorption, always take your fresh fruits and juices on an empty stomach and drink them as soon as they are ready. Leaving them to stand even for a minute will result in oxidation and wasted nourishment. Choose any quantity and ratio to suit your own appetite and taste.

GREAT JUICE MIXES

Apple and carrot
Apple and pear
Carrot, celery, watercress and any dark-leaved lettuce
Carrot, grape and apple
Celery, apple and carrot
Cucumber, beetroot and apple
Nectarine or peach with mango
Fresh pineapple and kiwi

LIVER CLEANSING JUICE

1 raw beetroot
1 small bunch of grapes
1 crisp apple

2 organic carrots
1 sprig of watercress

WONDERFUL WATER

No cleansing diet would work without water since toxins cannot be removed efficiently from a dehydrated system. Few people drink enough, even though most of us are aware that we need water for almost every single aspect of healthy function. It's still a common misconception that we need to drink water only when we're thirsty, and yet dehydration is considered to be a 'serious, frequent and costly medical problem', according to a report from The American Health Care Financing Administration. You don't just need extra fluid in hot weather or after workouts. If you work in an air-conditioned environment, you'll need more water. You also need to increase your fluid intake if you have a fever, respiratory infection or virus of any kind. Diets high in (usually hidden) salt also demand more fluid. It's worth knowing that, when we are born, our bodies are made up of 90 per cent water but, by the time we reach old age, content is down to around 60 per cent. A sobering thought! In a water-starved body, elimination of wastes slows down, cells suffocate and die in their own garbage! Keeping water intake high helps to keep the skin moist and firm and can actually hold back the ageing process!

I have found filtered water to be far superior to most bottled brands and certainly better than most tap water. A quality unit will remove a large proportion of heavy metals, chlorine and nitrates. Whatever brand you decide upon, write to manufacturers and ask to see independent test results before you buy. Don't give in to salesman hype! More information follows in Products and Services on page 357.

Use your filtered water every day whether you are detoxing or not – for drinking, cooking and filling the kettle.

Drink any water which is drained from vegetables after cooking. It will be rich in vitamins and minerals.

HELP YOUR DETOX ALONG BY SKIN BRUSHING

Healthy skin depends upon a healthy body. If the system is clogged and sluggish, new cells cannot work their way to the surface. Skin brushing stimulates the process of cell repair and renewal. Circulation is improved, impurities are released and skin is firmer, yet softer.

If your skin is too sensitive for a natural bristle skin brush, then use a towelling cloth, loofah or bath mitt. Stroke or brush – gently – towards the heart, beginning at the soles of the feet and working upwards. Make life more interesting by asking your partner to help!

Kathryn Marsden's book *Super Skin* contains lots more information on skin care and detoxification.

12

Eating for Energy: Increasing the Nutrients in Your Diet

'Because of their inadequate training in nutritional medicine and because of the natural delay in the clinical application of the new knowledge to individual patients, most doctors have difficulty in answering nutritional questions correctly. They often know no more than their patients – and sometimes even less.'

Dr Matti Tolonen
University of Helsinki

Increasing the variety of foods in the diet is an important part of beating fatigue. If we were absolutely honest, most of us would benefit from stretching our imagination a little, experimenting with new foods and knowing a bit more about where our nutrients come from.

If you thought that calcium was exclusive to cow's milk, that you lose out on Vitamin C if you don't drink orange juice or that the only place to find beta carotene is in carrots, the nutrient notes which begin on page 310 may surprise you. You'll find information on the best food sources of the most important vitamins and minerals together with information on those supplements which have a specific energy connection.

In the Food Sources lists you'll see that some items pop up more than once. For example, free-range eggs, fish, yoghurt, seeds, nuts, pulses, wholegrains, fruits and vegetables are all rich in a number of different nutrients. If your daily choices come from those groups, you're probably doing as well as you can in the healthy eating department. The lists are intended as a memory trigger, a reminder, to help you increase the variety of foods in your weekly shopping basket, perhaps invent a new dish or two and, in the process, improve your general nutrient intake.

SUPPLEMENTS FOR ENERGY

An increasing number of experts now agree that, although good food is an absolutely vital part of health maintenance, the hackneyed phrase 'you can get all the nutrients you need from a properly balanced diet' probably holds true for only a minority of the population. As the chapter on Energy and the Environment so clearly demonstrates, even those who follow the best of diets may still not be able to rely solely on their food to supply optimum nourishment or, for that matter, sufficient stamina and staying power.

Everything that happens in the body needs energy. We need it to fight illness, to repair and renew worn or damaged cells and to protect against a variety of different stressors; without energy we cannot walk, run, read, think or sleep; in essence, without a constant cache of internal energy, we just don't tick. To produce energy in the body – to keep the fire burning – we have to provide not just Calories but sufficient quantities of vitamins, minerals, enzymes, amino acids and essential fatty acids.

Unfortunately, a variety of hindrances such as pollution, ageing, inadequate diet, poor absorption and stress may prevent us from obtaining all we need for daily health maintenance. Indeed, it seems highly likely that, for a great many of us, the level of nourishment required for optimum wellbeing is just not getting through. In some cases – in illness or as a result of the ageing process perhaps – the body will use up the nutrients faster than they can be replaced; there may be insufficient nourishment in the basic diet or, possibly, the nutrients are being supplied but simply not being absorbed.

SCIENTIFIC BACK-UP

An estimated 10,000 papers are published each year on nutritional medicine and the use of specific vitamins, minerals, amino acids, essential fatty acids and herbs in the treatment of illness. Magnesium to reduce the risk of thrombosis after surgery and to help patients with osteoporosis, essential fatty acids in the treatment of skin disorders, vitamin E to improve heart function, vitamin B_{12} to help tinnitus, antioxidants to slow the progression of Parkinson's disease, garlic for improved circulation, zinc to improve fertility, vitamin A to enhance immunity, vitamin C to reduce recurring infections – these are just a few examples in a never-ending stream of positive data. Many studies confirm not only that multiple nutrient deficiencies are extremely widespread but also that diet alone may no longer be a reliable enough source of sustenance. Scurvy, beri-beri and rickets, common a century ago, may now be relatively rare but studies and surveys continue to demonstrate a worrying trend of missing or inadequate nutrients in the 'average' daily food supply. One has to wonder if the contemporaneous increase in difficult-to-define symptoms and not-so-good health is more than just a coincidence.

Despite mountains of research into the acknowledged link between deficiency disease and inadequate diet, the traditional view of most doctors remains that dietary supplements are quite unnecessary. But who says that the food we eat contains the right level of nourishment? How often are random samples of cauliflower, melon, banana or lamb's liver taken and tested to make sure they are nutritionally sound? Even if we had some domestic method of analysing every vitamin and every mineral in every foodstuff before we consumed it, such measurements give us no insight into how long the food was stored, whether or not there are any undesirable chemical residues involved, how much goodness was lost during preparation or the efficiency with which we absorb the meal in question.

TO SUPPLEMENT OR NOT TO SUPPLEMENT?

If you've had all the tests but nothing seems to fully explain why you've changed from a live wire into a burnt out fuse, then a three- to six-month course of carefully considered supplements could be the answer. I am not suggesting for a moment that it is necessary to take everything mentioned here. Nor is there any need to take large doses of several different products. There are products now available which will provide low doses of a balance of nutrients which act to 'top up' a good diet. Experience has shown that short term use (a few months, say) of some specific items can also be especially helpful in boosting flagging energy. For stockist details, see page 355.

First, re-assess your eating habits and try to obtain as much goodness as possible from your diet; then, if your health does not improve or you continue to feel chronically fatigued, excessively stressed or just not yourself, take advice on supplementation.

CO-Q10

When it comes to restoring energy, Co-Q10 (short for Co-enzyme Q10 and also called Ubiquinone or Vitamin Q) can pack a powerful punch. Co-Q10 is a co-enzyme which plays a vital role in the production of energy inside the cell. Without it, the body cannot extract energy from its power supply, in turn leaving us completely unable to function. A veritable mountain of research and other evidence has shown Q10 to be not only extremely safe but exceptionally effective for maintaining energy levels, improving heart function, keeping teeth and gums healthy, reducing the symptoms of the menopause, strengthening immunity and improving circulation. Although Co-Q10 is available to us in small amounts via our food supply, illness, ageing and poor liver function can affect the levels which we absorb. Taking a daily supplement of Co-Q10 has been likened to pouring petrol onto glowing embers.

Anyone wishing to read more about this fascinating substance may be interested in the book *Energy and Defense* by Gian Paolo Littarru. Details under Pharma Nord – page 355, Products and Services.

GINSENG *PANAX GINSENG*

Ginseng is well known as an *adaptogen*, something which has a normalizing, balancing action on the body. There is so much scientific research which confirms ginseng's ability to give anti-stress support to the adrenal system, to improve stamina and concentration and act as a general tonic that it is a difficult supplement to ignore. A three-month course to get you through a bad patch could be a good investment. Ginseng may also have anti-ageing and immune boosting properties.

Select with care, however. There are many types and grades of ginseng. The resulting quality will depend upon the age of the plant, where grown, which parts of the root are used and the method of extraction. If you choose a supplement which contains ginseng, then check the label for the words 'standardized' or 'guaranteed potency'. These terms indicate that the product has an assured level of active ingredients.

GINKGO BILOBA

The Ginkgo is believed to be the world's oldest tree, the one which Charles Darwin described as a 'living fossil'. Dinosaur fans may care to know that it was around during the Jurassic period – approximately 150 million years ago. Ginkgo biloba leaves contain several active properties including flavonoids which are known to strengthen blood vessels and capillaries and to improve circulation. Around 300 scientific studies have investigated Ginkgo biloba in relation to the circulation with latest investigations suggesting that the extract may also be of benefit in the relief of Raynaud's syndrome.

Research is now checking out Ginkgo biloba's apparent ability to mop up free radicals (molecules which, in excess, can cause cell damage) and to reduce allergic reactions and inflammation. As ginkgo is known to enhance oxygen transport and blood flow to the brain and to improve mental performance, it may also be a useful treatment for sufferers of Chronic Fatigue Syndrome, ME and anyone who has been sinking under mental (or physical) overload.

A great many other double blind trials have been carried out in which subjects reported improvements in short term memory, mood, emotional stability, depression, vertigo, headaches and respiratory ailments such as bronchitis and asthma.

As with ginseng, check that the produce you are buying contains 'standardized' extract. Take ginkgo according to the pack instructions for twelve to sixteen weeks and don't expect to see any results in less than 21–28 days. Studies show that the longer the treatment is continued, the more lasting are the results. Extensive toxicology studies have been carried out with this supplement. Apart from rare cases of mild gastrointestinal upset and mild headache, no toxicity was found.

OTHER FOOD SOURCES OF FLAVONOIDS

Apricots
Beetroot

Bilberries
Blackcurrants
Buckwheat
Cherries
Grapefruit peel and pulp
Grapes
Lemon peel and pulp
Cantaloup melon
Papaya
Green peppers

SILYMARIN

The herb *Silybum marianum* (often seen on product labels as Silymarin or Milk Thistle) is cleansing, regenerating, stimulating and protective to the liver. A short course of liver cleansing herbs can be a useful adjunct to treatment where there is lethargy, sluggishness, chronic fatigue, any kind of liver toxicity, skin complaints, arthritis, gall bladder problems, digestive disorders or candida. Practitioners also report Silymarin to be helpful in reducing the side effects of chemotherapy and in reducing the severity of asthma and hayfever.

ECHINACEA

The herb Echinacea deserves special mention in any book concerned with energy. Well-known for its immune-boosting properties and so valuable if you suffer from persistent infections, echinacea is also helpful where there is exhaustion and debility following illness.

LICORICE

Licorice (also on labels under its latin name, *Glycyrrhiza* or Liquorice) is another botanical worthy of consideration if you are treating long term lethargy or extreme exhaustion. From an energy point of view, licorice is supportive of the adrenal glands and the liver – two major players in the energy stakes.

You may find licorice, echinacea and milk thistle turning up together with added vitamins and minerals as a useful combination in some formulas.

THE B COMPLEX GROUP OF VITAMINS (including B_1, B_2, B_3, B_5, B_6, B_{12}, Folic acid, Biotin)

Food processing, freezing, insecticide sprays, sleeping drugs, the contraceptive pill, smoking and diets high in sugar are all likely to reduce the levels of B vitamins. The B group is well-known for its anti-stress action. If you are under excessive strain, feel generally run down, have a poor appetite, difficulty sleeping, hair, nail or skin problems or are unusually anxious or irritable, then a low-dose B Complex can offer valuable support.

Vitamin B_{12} deserves special mention. Although it is often included in B Complex supplements, my experience has been that a short course of B_{12} in addition to any regular daily B Complex or Multi Complex supplements can be very beneficial. (By the way, since most good Multivitamin products contain the B group, it shouldn't be necessary to take a B complex *and* a Multivitamin.)

Vitamin B_{12} works closely with folic acid, iron and vitamin C and is vital for a healthy nervous system and for the formation of red blood cells. This is a supplement worth considering (one tablet daily for a couple of months) if you are lethargic, anxious, stressed, depressed, generally run down or suffering from mental fatigue. Some ME sufferers have reported improved wellbeing after B_{12} injections. Studies also show that it might be a helpful supplement in multiple sclerosis, low blood pressure, asthma, hyperactivity and in elderly patients. The more obvious symptoms of deficiency are unusually pale skin, menstrual problems, fatigue, listlessness, 'jumpiness', swings of mood, twitchy limbs, poor co-ordination, tremors or a tongue which is abnormally red and smooth. If left untreated, B_{12} deficiency can lead to pernicious anaemia and degeneration of the nerve fibres in the spinal chord.

B vitamins are found in a wide range of foodstuffs. However, the best sources of B_{12} are found only in foods of animal origin; vegetarians and vegans should therefore consider a three-month course of tablets each year. Unlike iron, which can be toxic if it is supplemented unnecessarily, vitamin B_{12} is considered to be a very safe nutrient and can be used as a short-term general tonic even when there are no signs of clinical deficiency.

BEST FOOD SOURCES OF B VITAMINS

Apricots
Avocado

Bananas
Brown rice
Carrots
Chicken
Dried fruits
Free-range eggs
Grains
Lamb's kidney
Lamb's liver
Melon
Nuts
Oats
Oily fish
Pulses
Potatoes
Pumpkin
Root and green vegetables
Rye flour
Salad produce
Soya flour
Spirulina (a nutritious algae and one of the few plant
          sources of vitamin B12)
Yoghurt

VITAMIN C

Another important anti-stress nutrient which is easily
wiped out by smoking, car exhaust fumes and other pollutants, vitamin C is also a powerful antioxidant and
detoxifier. When taken daily, vitamin C appears to
reduce the risk of viral attack. Extra vitamin C can

also reduce the severity of cold and flu symptoms and speed recovery time. A human suffering any kind of stress will use up large quantities of vitamin C – a fact which may go some way towards explaining why people under stress seem more likely to 'catch' colds and flu. As explained in the chapters on Sleep and Energy and the Environment, it can be an extremely wise health insurance to take extra vitamin C every day, whatever your health status. If you are subjected regularly to any kind of pollution, vitamin C becomes even more important. Look on the label for the words 'low acid formula', 'buffered' or 'ascorbate'; these complexes tend to be more easily absorbed and less likely to upset the digestion than cheaper brands of plain ascorbic acid.

BEST FOOD SOURCES OF VITAMIN C

Most fresh vegetable and fruit produce should contain some vitamin C. These are some of the best sources:

Blackcurrants
Broccoli
Brussels sprouts
Cabbage
Cauliflower
Acerola cherries – West Indian cherries – a type particularly rich in vitamin C
Grapefruits
Kale
Kiwi fruit
Lemons
Mustard & Cress

Parsley
Green and red peppers
Rosehips
Sweet potatoes
Tomatoes
Watercress

I have not included oranges in this list as both the fruit and the juice can cause allergic reactions and stomach pain in some people.

IRON

This nutrient should be treated with respect. Iron deficiency is believed to be one of the most widespread deficiencies of all nutrients and, yet, indiscriminate supplementation of iron can be dangerous. As explained on page 155, the best answer probably is to make certain your diet contains a varied list of iron-rich foods but to avoid iron supplements unless your doctor has advised that you need extra iron.

BEST FOOD SOURCES OF IRON

Asparagus
Blackstrap molasses
Dark green vegetable and salad foods
Dried fruit
Free-range eggs
Green and red peppers
Lamb's liver
Oatmeal

Parsley
Pulses
Seafood
Watercress

Interesting to note that quite a number of foods which contain vitamin C also contain iron. Iron absorption is enhanced if vitamin C is taken at the same time.

SELENIUM

Selenium is another example of the fascinating paradox that something which is dangerously toxic in excess can be extremely therapeutic in sensible doses. There are a number of studies which show that this trace mineral is capable of detoxifying heavy metals such as mercury, lead and cadmium. One of the earliest signs of heavy metal toxicity is fatigue. Selenium is also a powerful antioxidant and may have a role to play in reducing the incidence of cancer, arthritis and heart disease. Intensive farming, over-used soil and food processing can all reduce the levels of selenium found in food. Anyone who has mercury amalgam in their teeth should take extra selenium as should anyone who works with smokers or lives or travels in a polluted environment. Selenium is found as part of most quality Multi Complexes or Antioxidant Complexes and so is not usually needed as a separate supplement.

BEST FOOD SOURCES OF SELENIUM

Broccoli
Fish

Free-range eggs
Garlic
Lamb's kidney
Lamb's liver
Onions
Shellfish
Tomatoes
Wholegrains – especially brown rice

CHROMIUM

As chromium is an important trace element needed for proper blood glucose balance and insulin production (see page 171), a deficiency of it can quickly lead to fatigue, hypoglycaemia and, possibly, even diabetes. Studies show that chromium is commonly deficient in the average diet but is also susceptible to crop spraying and food processing. If you are troubled by food cravings and symptoms of hypoglycaemia and a check-up can find nothing else wrong, increase your intake of chromium-rich foods and consider a short course (3–6 months) of chromium supplementation either in liquid or capsule form. If chromium is already included in your daily Multicomplex, then it should not be necessary to take the mineral separately.

BEST FOOD SOURCES OF CHROMIUM:

Asparagus
Beetroot (raw)

Blackstrap molasses
Cheese
Chicken
Egg yolk
Lamb's liver
Sea vegetables
Seafood
Spirulina

MAGNESIUM

Magnesium acts as a co-enzyme in a number of energy-producing processes throughout the body; it helps in the efficient function of vitamins B_1 and B_6, calcium, potassium and sodium and is vital for healthy hormonal and nervous systems. There is much encouraging evidence that magnesium could also be an important nutrient in the treatment and relief of stress, exhaustion, ME and Chronic Fatigue Syndrome (see page 210). Courses of magnesium (by injection or as oral supplements) may be particularly useful in relieving pain, fatigue and spasm in muscles. However, not all magnesium products are of equal quality. For example, there are reports of magnesium oxide causing stomach upset and diarrhoea and of magnesium carbonate triggering attacks of indigestion. Anyone considering the use of magnesium supplements should check product labels carefully and seek advice from a qualified practitioner who has nutritional experience.

BEST FOOD SOURCES OF MAGNESIUM

- Apples
- Bananas
- Brown rice
- Dried fruits – especially figs
- Fish
- Ginger root
- Grains
- Grapefruit
- Green vegetables
- Lamb
- Lemons
- Nuts, i.e. almonds, Brazils, cashews
- Pasta
- Pulses
- Seafood

CALCIUM

Calcium is ubiquitous in our food supply. So many different foods contain varying amounts of this mineral that, in a varied diet, it should be possible to obtain the right calcium levels from food sources alone (see list below) – even if milk is removed from the diet. Anyone experiencing persistent lack of energy should consider cutting down on cow's milk. This common allergen is not only mucus-forming for many people but also can be difficult to digest. Small quantities added to tea or coffee are less of a problem but large amounts are not recommended.

An overload of calcium from unnecessary supplements may do more harm than good. This does not mean that calcium is bad for us – far from it. However, it may be more sensible to keep your calcium reserves topped up from your food supply than from tablets or milk. If you have a family history of osteoporosis or are worried about brittle bone disease, see your GP for a check-up and ask to be referred to a nutrition practitioner. An increasing number of reports now suggest that it may be more valuable to supplement magnesium than calcium, especially where there are bone disorders.

BEST FOOD SOURCES OF CALCIUM

Brown rice
Buttermilk
Canned salmon
Canned sardines
Cheese
Figs
Nuts, i.e. almonds and Brazils
Oats
Pulses
Sea vegetables – available in dried form from health food stores; ideal for adding extra flavour to stews, casseroles and soups
Stock made with bones
Sunflower seeds, sesame seeds, tahini
Tofu
Yoghurt
The majority of vegetables and herbs contain some

calcium. Especially good sources are okra, kale, parsley, watercress, dandelion leaves, broccoli, vine leaves, taro leaves, onions, fenugreek, drumstick leaves, cabbage, Brussels sprouts, parsnip, turnip, turnip tops, carrot and swede. It's worth knowing that roots and stalks are particularly rich in this mineral.

ESSENTIAL FATTY ACIDS (EFAs)

Although available from food sources, some scientists believe that many of us may no longer have the facility to convert the EFAs in food into usable substances within the system. One way to overcome the problem is to supplement. Several reports suggest that increasing intake of essential fatty acids can reduce fatigue, increase energy levels and boost immune function. The best way to increase your intake of EFAs is to eat more oily fish, take a tablespoon of linseeds each day with a glass of water, eat plenty of other seeds and nuts (not peanuts) as well as a wide variety of vegetables. Those with suspected or diagnosed ME or Chronic Fatigue Syndrome, recurring infections, hormonal imbalances, skin disorders or problems with circulation should try a six-month course of either GLA (gamma linolenic acid) or evening primrose oil. It's worth knowing that supplements do not produce overnight results and improvements may not be seen for anything from 12 to 16 weeks.

BEST NATURAL SOURCES OF ESSENTIAL FATTY ACIDS

Cold-pressed oils
Evening primrose oil
GLA supplements
Oily fish
Nuts
Seeds

BEST FOOD SOURCES OF MANGANESE

Almonds
Avocado
Bananas
Raw beetroot
Blackberries
Brazils
Chestnuts
Coconut
Dark leaved lettuce
Egg yolk
Green leafy vegetables
Hazelnuts
Cold-pressed honey
Oats
Olives
Peas
Pineapple
Rye bread

BEST FOOD SOURCES OF POTASSIUM

Coffee, tea
   and grain-based beverages
Dried fruits
Fresh fruits and juices
Garlic
Ginger root
Grains
Molasses
Muesli
Potatoes
Salad and vegetable produce
Soya flour

BEST FOOD SOURCES OF ZINC

Cheese
Crab
Fish
Free-range eggs
Lamb chops
Lamb's liver
Meat
Pumpkin seeds
Sea vegetables
Shrimps

BEST FOOD SOURCES OF BETA CAROTENE

Most fresh green, red and yellow/orange produce, including:

Apricots
Asparagus
Broccoli
Butter
Cantaloup melon
Carrots
Cashew nuts
Cauliflower greens
Cheese
Cream
Nectarines
Parsley
Peaches
Green peppers
Pumpkin
Spinach
Spring greens
Sweet potatoes
Turnip tops
Watercress

BEST FOOD SOURCES OF VITAMIN A

Butter
Cheese
Cod liver oil

328

Free-range eggs
Halibut liver oil
Lamb's liver
Oily fish

BEST FOOD SOURCES OF VITAMIN E

Oils (cold-pressed oils only), especially:
Cod liver
Extra virgin olive
Linseed
Rice bran
Safflower
Soya bean
Sunflower
Also:
Apples
Bananas
Broccoli
Brown rice
Brussels sprouts
Carrots
Cashew nuts
Free-range eggs
Grains
Granola
Lamb's liver
Nuts
Onions
Potatoes
Salmon

Seeds
Shrimps
Soya beans
Spinach

BEST FOOD SOURCES OF VITAMIN D

Cod liver oil
Free-range eggs
Mackerel
Salmon
Sardines
Tuna

Vitamin D is also produced by the action of ultra violet light on the skin.

A SPECIAL SUPPLEMENT: GARCINIA CAMBOGIA

When a body is a bit overweight, good dietary management and regular exercise, if followed sensibly, should be sufficient to bring that weight under control. For those with ongoing weight problems, food combining has also been shown to be an extremely safe and effective way to shed excess pounds. However, for anyone who is plagued by stubborn weight which just won't move, a new supplement – extracted from the fruit Garcinia cambogia – may be helpful. May I stress, however, that this is not something that should be used by anyone who is trying to lose a mere pound or two. Garcinia cambogia is available without prescription but should be used only following medical advice and, preferably, under practitioner supervision in conjunction with a healthy eating programme. Supplier details are on page 355.

> A word of caution: I would reiterate my earlier recommendation that anyone with an energy problem first takes medical advice and keeps their GP informed of any dietary changes they are making. Supplements are not meal replacements or substitutes for proper rest, relaxation or healthy eating habits. They can, however, offer welcome support to a tired, exhausted and run-down system. Follow the pack instructions and do not take more than the recommended dose. Small, measured amounts can be stimulating, uplifting and energizing. Excesses of *anything* can be dangerous.

SOURCES OF REFERENCE:

Semba R D, Ward B J. Abnormal T Cell Subset Proportions in Vitamin A Deficient Children. *Lancet* 1993;341:5–8.
England M R, Gordon G, Salem M, Chernow B. Magnesium administration and dysrhythmias after cardiac surgery: a placebo controlled, double-blind, randomized trial. *Journal of the American Medical Association* 1992;268:2395–2402.
Abraham G E. The Importance of Magnesium in the

Management of Primary Postmenopausal Osteoporosis. *Journal of Nutritional Medicine* 1991;2:165–8.

Woods K L, Fletcher S, Roffe C, Haider Y. Intravenous magnesium sulphate in suspected acute myocardial infarction: results of the second Leicester Intravenous Magnesium Intervention Trial. *Lancet* 1992;39:1553–8.

Vikkanski L. Magnesium may slow bone loss. *Medical Tribune* 1993;22 July;page 9.

Buist, R. Ginkgo biloba – an in-depth report. *Blackmores Communicator* 1993;3(7):1–2.

Ginkgo. Kew Information Sheet 06. Kindly provided by the Royal Botanical Gardens, Kew.

Middleton E et al. Naturally occurring flavonoids and human basophil histamine release. *Archives of Allergy and Applied Immunology* 1985;77:155–7.

Kleijnen J, Knipschild P. Ginkgo Biloba. *Lancet* 1992;340:1124–7.

Houghton P. Ginkgo. *The Pharmaceutical Journal* 1994;253:122–3.

Vitamin B_{12} – Powerful Protection Against Asthma. Author unknown. Article published in *International Clinical Nutritional Review* 1989;9(4):185–88.

Anibarro B, Caballero T, Garcia-Ara C, Diaz-Pena J M, Ojeda J A. Asthma with sulfite intolerance in children: a blocking study with cyanocobalamin. *Journal of Allergy and Clinical Immunology* 1991;90:103–9.

Newbold H L. Vitamin B_{12} – Placebo or neglected therapeutic tool. *Medical Hypotheses* 1989;28:155–64.

Lossos A, Argov Z. Orthostatic hypotension induced by vitamin B_{12} deficiency. *Journal of the American Geriatric Society* 1991;39:601–3.

Yao Y et al. Prevalence of vitamin B_{12} deficiency among geriatric outpatients. *Journal of the Family Practitioner* 1992;35:524–8.

Unrecognized cobalamin-responsive neuropsychiatric disorders. Editorial. *Nutrition Review* 1989;47(7):208–10. Also reported in *International Clinical Nutrition Review* April 1990.

Notes taken from the Seventh and Eighth International Symposia on The Biochemical and Clinical Aspects of Coenzyme Q. Copenhagen, Denmark: 18–19 September 1992; Stockholm, Sweden: 11–13 November 1993.

Vitamins and Minerals in Health and Nutrition by M. Tolonen, Ellis Horwood/Van Nostrand-Reinhold, 1990.

Energy and Defense by Gian Pasto Li Haru, Casa Editrice Scientifica Internazionale.

13

Twelve Top Tips for Lifting Energy

After reading all this information about energy, you must be feeling exhausted! Turn to these top twelve tips whenever you're flagging and need encouragement.

1. For best energy reserves, eat protein foods earlier in the day and keep the carbohydrates for the evening. Whilst carbos are calming and can help you to wind down at the end of the day, proteins can kick your brain into gear and may even help to lift your mood.

2. Avoid these energy gobblers: wheat-based bread and breakfast cereals, yeast, cow's milk and sugar. Read the labels! Then check pages 284–285 for more details.

3. However busy you are, allocate a few minutes each day for exercise. A brisk walk in the fresh air is enough to maintain that feel good factor.

4. Breathe more deeply. Stretch and yawn. Rub the backs of your hands and the soles of your feet. Massage gently but firmly around the ear lobes.

5. Eat regular meals. Don't miss out because you think that cutting a whole load of calories is a quick fix remedy for staying slim. It isn't. And don't become a professional dieter. Extreme calorie counting is the quickest way to encourage an energy slump.

6. Don't go all day without food only to binge on a huge meal in the evening. Eating little and often makes for more efficient digestion and puts more nutrients in the energy store cupboard.

7. It makes sense to cut down on the hidden fat found in energy-sapping processed foods such as ready made meals, packets and tins, cakes and cookies. But don't reduce fat intake too far. Although excess fat is believed to encourage heart disease, too little can do the same. The right kinds and amounts of fat can give us essential vitamins and fatty acids not found in abundance elsewhere and is also a source of, guess what? . . . energy.

8. Include plenty of variety in your diet. It you are stuck on only a few foods – even if they are in the rabbit food category, your nourishment rate is likely to be low, your energy rating even lower.

9. Beware of overdoing the beverage buzz. Coffee, tea and cola should be no problem for most people as long as these are used sensibly and in moderation but load up the caffeine and you can feel wiped out later. Drink more water, preferably filtered or bottled.

10. Take a break from what you are doing. A change of scene, even for a few minutes, can give your energy a lift.

11. Explore different food combinations. Simple food combining can make a real difference to energy levels because of the way in which it improves digestion. Fall back on food combining whenever you need an energy boost. Don't restrict portion sizes or count calories. Eat until you are comfortably full. Follow the 'don't mix proteins with starches' rule during the week and then forget it at weekends.

12. Top up your healthy diet with a simple supplement programme that contains protective antioxidants and the new energy helper Co-Enzyme Q10.

Health check: If your energy lows are not responding or you are concerned in any way about your health, ask your GP for a check up. Deficiencies of iron or Vitamin B$_{12}$, very high or very low blood pressure, over- or under-active thyroid are just a few of the health problems which cause tiredness.

HEALTHY EATER SWAP BOX

SWAP	FOR
Pork and beef	Fresh fish, free-range poultry and lean lamb
Battery and barn eggs	Free-range eggs
Cow's milk	Yoghurt
Deep frying	Stir-frying, grilling, & casseroles
The chip pan	A steamer and a wok
Hydrogenated spreads	A little butter
Any cooking oil	Extra virgin olive oil
Take-aways	Doing it yourself
Readymade meals	Use the fresh versions; they're more nourishing and just as quick to prepare
Crisps & peanuts	Pumpkin & sunflower seeds, almonds, pecans, Brazils, hazelnuts & macadamias
Chocolate	Dried fruit, especially figs; choose organic chocolate for treats
Sugar	Cold pressed honey
Chips	Organic jacket potatoes

---

continued

Ordinary bread	Yeast-free bread, rice cakes, rye bread, pumpernickel (black rye), oatcakes
White flour, white rice white pasta	Use the brown version — sorry, this doesn't include sugar
Packet cereals	Make your own from oats, seeds, nuts & dried fruit

Further Reading

HIGHLY RECOMMENDED

Love is Letting Go of Fear by Gerald G. Jampolsky MD, Celestial Arts, California.
Worth it for the cartoons alone but a great collection of common sense and affirmations to nurture peace of mind. Based on *A Course in Miracles*, transcribed by William Thetford and Helen Schucman, Foundation for Inner Peace.

Frontiers of Health by Dr Christine Page, C W. Daniel.
For anyone interested in the mind/body connection and how emotions can contribute to disease. A stunning book – don't read it if you don't want to read about yourself.

Stop the Insanity by Susan Powter, Orion Books.
It is impossible not to admire Susan Powter – for her determination, her humour and her common sense. This book is aimed primarily at those who have suffered at the hands of the diet food and fitness industries but is well worthwhile for anyone who enjoys a good read and needs to laugh.

Meditations for Women Who Do Too Much by Anne Wilson Schaef, Harper San Francisco.
A collection of the most wonderful observations, meditations and affirmations. Essential reading for all exhausted women.

Peace, Love and Healing by Bernie Siegel, Rider/ Century Hutchinson.

The second Siegel bestseller. Written originally for cancer patients and their families, it is an essential read for anyone whatever their health status. Funny, interesting and immensely helpful.

What Doctors Don't Tell You (WDDTY), 4 Wallace Road, London, N1 2PG. Twelve issues yearly. Send stamped addressed envelope or airmail coupons for details. Subscriptions available worldwide. Essential information on what really goes on behind medical/surgical scenes, up-to-date drug research and details of side effects plus valuable alternative treatments.

WDDTY also produce booklets on specific subjects; for example, 'Guide to Candida and ME', 'A Guide to the Dangers of Fillings and Fluoride' and 'How to be an Assertive Patient'. Highly recommended.

AROMATHERAPY

Aromatherapy for the Family by Jan Kusmirek (a pocket booklet available from The Institute of Classical Aromatherapy, 17 The Crescent, Taunton, Somerset TA1 4EB. £1.25 including postage and packing).

The Aromatherapy Handbook by Daniele Ryman, C W. Daniel.

Aromatherapy for You at Home by Franzesca Watson (available from Natural by Nature Oils Ltd, The Aromatherapy Centre, 9 Vivian Avenue, Hendon Central, London NW4 3UT. £2.50 including postage and packing).

Aromatherapy – A guide for home use by Christine Westwood, Amberwood Publishing.
Aromantics by Valerie Ann Worwood, Bantam Books.
The Fragrant Pharmacy by Valerie Ann Worwood, Bantam Books.

COLOUR

Healing Through Colour by Theo Gimbel, C W. Daniel.
Colour Me Beautiful by Carole Jackson, Piatkus Books.
Frontiers of Health by Dr Christine R Page, C W. Daniel.
The Healing Power of Colour by Betty Wood, Aquarian Press.

ENVIRONMENT

The New House Plant Expert by David Hessayon, Expert Books.
Radiation Protection Manual by Dr Lita Lee (available from Grassroots Network, 2061 Hampton Avenue, Redwood City CA 94061, USA; $6.95 plus postage. Please check with supplier re overseas mailing costs).
The Natural House by David Pearson, Gaia.

FOOD

Food: An Oxford Anthology edited by Brigid Allen, Oxford University Press.

Berrydales Special Diet News edited by Michelle Berriedale-Johnson (available on subscription from Berrydale Publishers, Berrydale House, 5 Lawn Road, London NW3 2XS. Contains extremely useful information on special diets and is particularly valuable to those with allergies and food sensitivities. Please send s.a.e. for information).

French Vegetarian Cookery by Paola Gavin, Optima.

How to Dine Like the Devil and Feel Like a Saint by Luc De Schepper (available from Full of Life Publishing, 500 N. Guadalupe St, G441 Santa Fe, New Mexico 87501, USA; $20.25. Please check with the suppliers re overseas mailing costs).

GEOPATHIC STRESS

Are You Sleeping in a Safe Place by Rolf Gordon (write to him, care of 130 Gypsy Hill, London SE19 1PL; £5.95 post free UK, £8.50 overseas).

HERBAL REMEDIES

The Hamlyn Guide to Edible and Medicinal Plants by Edmund Launert, Hamlyn.

The A–Z of Modern Herbalism by Simon Y. Mills, Thorsons.

The Herb Bible by Earl Mindell, Vermilion.

The Complete Woman's Herbal by Anne McIntyre, Gaia.

HORMONES

Sexual Chemistry – Understanding our Hormones, the Pill and HRT by Dr Ellen Grant, Cedar Mandarin.
Balance Hormones Naturally by Kate Neil, ION.

HYPNOTHERAPY

Self-Hypnosis by Valerie Austin, Thorsons.

POSTURE/REDUCING STRESS AT WORK

Are You Sitting Comfortably? by Andrew Wilson, Optima.

RELAXATION/MEDITATION/VISUALIZATION

Creative Visualization by Shakti Gawain, Bantam Books.
Stress Busters by Robert Holden, Thorsons.
How to Meditate by Lawrence LeShan, Crucible/Turnstone Press.
The Calm Technique by Paul Wilson, Thorsons.

THYROID TREATMENT

Hypothyroidism: The Unsuspected Illness by Broda Barnes and Lawrence Galton, Harper & Row.

The Broda Barnes Research Foundation, PO Box 98, Trumbull, Connecticut 06611, USA, is a research organization involved in thyroid research. If you write to them for information, please send international reply coupons with your self-addressed envelope.

WHERE TO FIND PRODUCTS AND SERVICES

When writing to any of these addresses, please offer the courtesy of a stamped-addressed envelope or international reply coupons. Several of the companies listed here will supply worldwide.

AROMATHERAPY PRODUCTS

Aromatherapy oils are available at most good chemists, health food stores and by mail order. For additional information contact:

Gerard House, 475 Capability Green, Luton, Bedfordshire LU1 3LU. Telephone: 01582 487331. (From health food stores).

Natural by Nature Oils Ltd, 9 Vivian Avenue, Hendon Central, London NW4 3UT. Telephone: 0181 202 5718. (Mail order and health food stores. Natural by Nature Oils also offer training courses in aromatherapy massage.)

Natural Image Ltd, Ashby House, Bath Street, Ashby-de-la-Zouch, Leics. LE65 2FH. Telephone: 01530 563900. (Mail order.)

Nelson Homoeopathic Pharmacy, 73 Duke Street, Grosvenor Square, London, W1M 6BY. Telephone: 0171 495 2404. (Mail order.)

AUSTRALIA

In Essence Aromatherapy, 3 Abbott Street, Fairfield, Vic 3078. Telephone: (03) 497 1411.

Sunspirit Oils Pty Ltd, 6 Ti-tree Place, Byron Bay, NSW 2481. Telephone: (066) 856 333.

Absolute Essential Ltd, 93 College Hill, Ponsonby, Auckland. Telephone: (09) 360 0914. (Mail order available).
The Oil Company – Bespoke Aromatherapy Ltd, PO Box 3454, Auckland. Telephone: (09) 522 0416. (Mail order available).

ENVIRONMENT

The Soil Association, 86 Colston Street, Bristol, Avon BS1 5BB. Telephone: 0117 9290661. Regional Guides available giving information relating to stockists, opening times, types of produce sold, delivery and mail order services county by county.
The National Society for Clean Air, 136, North Street, Brighton, East Sussex BN1 1RG. Send s.a.e. for information leaflets and membership details.
Amway. Suppliers of environmentally-friendly household cleaning products, also rebounder equipment (mini-trampoline). For details of nearest distributor, write to Amway Information Centre, Snowdon Drive, Winterhill, Milton Keynes, Bucks MK6 1AR. Telephone: 01908 679888. Amway products are available worldwide.
The Little Green Shop, 16 Gardner Street, Brighton, East Sussex, BN1 1UP. Telephone: 01273 571221.

Household products suitable for allergy sufferers and those sensitive to chemicals. Please send large s.a.e. or international reply coupons for mail order catalogue.

Nutshell Supplies, Newlake Cottage, Staverton, Devon TQ9 6PE. Telephone/Fax: 01803 762329. Suppliers of mineral and plant-based household paints, oils, polish, wood preservatives, etc. Suitable for allergy sufferers and those sensitive to chemicals. Please send large s.a.e. for mail order catalogue.

The National Bed Federation Ltd, 251 Brompton Road, London SW3 2EZ. Telephone: 0171 589 4888. Very useful self-help guide to cutting down the risk of allergy.

The Radon Survey, National Radiological Protection Board, Chilton, Didcot, Oxfordshire OX11 0RQ.

The Women's Environmental Network, Aberdeen Studios, 22 Highbury Grove, London N5 2EA. Telephone: 0171 354 8823. For those interested in keeping up to date with environmental issues. Send large s.a.e. for details. Membership available.

Naturcare panty shields, press-on towels, etc. Non-chlorine bleach, plastic-free products; kinder to the environment. For stockist details, write to Bodywise (UK) Ltd, 14 Lower Court Road, Lower Almondsbury, Bristol BS12 4DX.

If you are concerned about animal welfare and factory farming and are interested in supporting and receiving information from non-violent pressure groups, contact:

Compassion in World Farming (CIWF), 5A Charles Street, Petersfield, Hampshire GU32 3EH, England, or CIWF, PO Box 206, Cork, Ireland for their

Action Pack and membership details. CIWF also have a youth group called FarmWatch.

also

Farm Animal Welfare Network, PO Box 40, Holmfirth, Huddersfield, West Yorkshire HD7 1QY, England.

AUSTRALIA

Total Environment Centre, (& Toxic Chemicals Committee), 1/88 Cumberland Street, Sydney, NSW 2000. Telephone: (02) 247 4714.

The Cleanhouse Effect, 345 King Street, Newtown, NSW 2042. Telephone: (02) 516 4681.

Amway Distributors Australia Wide, 46 Carrington Road, Castle Hill, NSW 2154. Telephone: (02) 843 2000.

EXERCISE

The Exercise Association, Unit 4, Angel Gate, City Road, London EC1V 2PT. Please send a large s.a.e. for information.

Active Lifestyle magazine, 41 Overstone Road, London W6 0PH. Produced bimonthly – from newsagents or by subscription. In case of difficulty, write to them enclosing s.a.e.

FOOD SUPPLIERS

First Class Foods, PO Box 30, Daventry, Northants NN11 4US. Telephone: 01327 300502. Fax: 01327 310528.

Tea and Coffee. Better quality teas and coffees tend to be naturally lower in caffeine without the need to use decaffeinated products. For information, price list and mail order supplies, contact **Kendricks Coffee Company,** Tea and Coffee Specialists, Ocean Parade, South Ferring, Worthing, West Sussex, BN12 5QQ. Telephone: 01903 503244.

GEOPATHIC STRESS

What Doctors Don't Tell You (WDDTY), 4 Wallace Road, London, N1 2PG. Information available on power lines and electro-magnetic pollution. Send a stamped addressed envelope or airmail coupons for further details. Subscriptions are available worldwide. *What Doctors Don't Tell You* also offers essential information on specific subjects related to health and well-being. Highly recommended.

Dowser/Kinesiologist; Jacqueline Beacon; Telephone: 0181 455 7912. Distant dowsing and assistance by telephone.

Sabona copper bracelets. Available by mail order and in some selected outlets. For details, write to Sabona at 4 Blythe Mews, Blythe Road, London W14 0HW. Telephone: 0171 603 0656.

The following specialists undertake environmental surveys into electromagnetic radiation and geopathic stress:

Bill Jackson, 14 Farm Street, Speers Point, NSW 2284. Telephone: (049) 584000.
Victor & Edith Knobloch, Adelaide, SA. Telephone: (08) 339 5716.
Rhona Khoury, 43 Hansens Road, Minto Heights, NSW 2566.Telephone: (02) 603 3369.

NEW ZEALAND
Albino Gola, 39 Ellerton Road, Mt.Eden, Auckland 1003. Telephone: (09) 638 8622.

HOMOEOPATHIC REMEDIES

Homoeopathic medicines are available from health food stores and by mail from Ainsworths Homoeopathic Pharmacy, 38 New Cavendish Street, London W1M 9FG. Telephone 0171 935 5330. Talk to Ainsworths about their homoeopathic travel packs and first-aid remedies, especially if you are travelling abroad.
For Nelson Homoeopathic Pharmacy see under Aromatherapy.

AUSTRALIA
Brauer, 1 Para Road, Tanunda, SA 5352. National Freecall Advisory Line: 1800 008 108 (within Australia).

JUICING EQUIPMENT

Braun UK Ltd, Dolphin Estate, Windmill Road, Sunbury-on-Thames, Middlesex TW16 7EJ. Telephone: 01932 785611.

AUSTRALIA
Braun (Australia) Pty Ltd, Private Bag 917, N Sydney Shopping World Post Office, NSW 2060. Freecall 008 656808 (within Australia).

ME

Action for ME, PO Box 1302, Wells, Somerset BA5 2WE. Please send a large s.a.e. for their very helpful information pack. Action for ME also have two telephone helplines. Call either 01749 670799 or the 24-hour recorded information service on 0891 122976. Remember that 0891 numbers attract higher call rates.
ME Association, Stanhope House, High Street, Stanford-le-Hope, Essex SS17 0HA. Please send s.a.e.

AUSTRALIA
ME/Chronic Fatigue Syndrome Society, PO Box 449, Crows Nest, NSW 2065. Telephone: (02) 439 6026.

NEW ZEALAND
ANZME Society, PO Box 36307, Northcote, Auckland.

NON-HYDROGENATED SPREADS

Vitaquell is available from most health food stores. Further details from the UK Distributors, Brewhurst Health Food Supplies, Abbot Close, Oyster Lane, Byfleet, Surrey KT14 7JP. Telephone: 01932 354211.

AUSTRALIA
Vital, an Australian lecithin spread, and all nut butters are non-hydrogenated and are available from health food stores and selected supermarkets.

HOW TO FIND A PRACTITIONER

The following UK-based organizations hold lists of registered practitioners:

The Institute for Complementary Medicine (ICM), PO Box 194, London SE16 1QZ. Telephone: 0171 237 5175.

The National Federation of Spiritual Healers, will provide you with the name of a healer in your area. Call them on 01891 616080.

The Register of Chinese Herbal Medicine, PO Box 400, Wembley, Middlesex HA9 9NZ. Please send s.a.e.

The Register of Traditional Chinese Medicine, 19 Trinity Road, London N2 8JJ. Please send s.a.e.

The International Register of Oriental Medicine, 4 The Manor House, Coley Lane, Reigate, Surrey RH2 9JW. Please send s.a.e.

A few hospitals now offer Chinese medicine. Check with your GP or local Family Health Service Authority (in the phone book).

The British Chiropractic Association, 29 Whitley Street, Reading, Berkshire RG2 0EG. Send s.a.e. or phone 01734 757557.

The McTimoney Chiropractic School, 14 Park End Street, Oxford OX1 1HH. Send s.a.e. or phone 01865 246786.

The UK Homoeopathic Medical Association, 6 Livingston Road, Gravesend, Kent DA12 5DZ. Please send s.a.e.

If you live in London, the following multi-therapy centres offer a wide range of services and valuable information:
All Hallows House, Idol Lane, London EC3R 5DD. Telephone: 0171 283 8908.

The Hale Clinic, 7 Park Crescent, London W1N 3HE. Telephone: 0171 631 0156.

For further study information contact:
The Raworth Centre, 20-26 South Street, Dorking, Surrey RH4 2HQ. Telephone: 01306 742150.

I.O.N., Blades Court, Deodar Road, London SW15 2NU. Telephone: 0181 877 9993.

AUSTRALIA

Call: Blackmores Naturopathic Clinic, Balgowlah, Sydney, (02) 948 5653, or House of Blackmores, Victoria, (03) 853 0056, or Blackmores (Australia-wide), 008 803 760.

Australian Traditional Medicine Society, PO Box 442, Ryde, NSW 2112. Telephone: (02) 809 6800. (Directory of practitioners includes Naturopathy, Homoeopathy,

Herbal Medicine, Nutrition, Acupuncture, Chinese
Herbal Medicine and Massage Therapies).
**Australian College of Nutritional & Environmental
Medicine**, 13 Hilton Street, Beaumaris, Vic 3193.
Telephone: (03) 589 6088.

For further study information contact:
**Nature Care, College of Naturopathic & Traditional
Medicine,**1A Frederick Street, Artarmon, NSW 2064.
Telephone: (02) 439 8844.
(Diploma and Certificated Courses offered in
Aromatherapy, Reflexology, Shiatsu, Nutrition,
Homoeopathy, Herbal Medicine, Remedial Massage,
Naturopathy, plus many short courses).

NEW ZEALAND
Call: **Blackmores**, (09) 415 8585.
South Pacific Association of Natural Therapists, 68
Wellpark Avenue, Westmere, Auckland. Telephone:
(09) 360 0560.

SAD

Full Spectrum Lighting Ltd, Unit 1, Riverside
Business Centre, Victoria Street, High Wycombe,
Buckinghamshire HP11 2LT. Telephone: 01494 526051
or 448727. Suppliers of full spectrum lighting boxes,
bulbs and tubes.
In Scotland: **F.S.I. Scotland**, Unit 11, 42 Dalsetter

Avenue, Glasgow G15 8SL. Telephone: 0141 944 2647.
The SAD Association, PO Box 989, London SW7 2PZ.
also:
Chrystal Branch, Ashridge, Desborough Road, Rushton,
Kettering, Northamptonshire NN14 1RG. Mrs Branch is
an ex-sufferer and adviser on Seasonal Affective Disorder.

AUSTRALIA
Phillips Australia produce triphosphor tubes (TLD
colour 80 & TLD colour 90) which are available through
electrical wholesalers.

SUPPLEMENT SUPPLIERS

Blackmores – Herbals (including passiflora and valerian), vitamins, minerals, antioxidants and acidophilus.
Also supplements containing Co-Q10, chromium, B
complex, ginkgo and ginseng. From health food stores. In
case of difficulty, contact Blackmores Ltd, Unit 7 Poyle
Tech Centre, Willow Road, Poyle, Colnbrook, Bucks LS3
0PD. Telephone: 01753 683815.
Pharma Nord – Co-Q10, antioxidants and other products. Should be available from good health food stores.
Contact Pharma Nord (UK) Ltd, Spital Hall, Mitford,
Morpeth, Northumberland NE61 3PN. Telephone:
01670 519989. The Co-Q10 book, *Energy and Defense*, is
available direct from Pharma Nord.
Biocare – Garcinia cambogia, Jetzyme anti-jet stress
enzymes, multivitamins and minerals, GLA, acidophilus,
anti-fungals, artemesia, liquid chromium, B complex,
antioxidants and vitamin C. Mail order only from Biocare

Ltd, 54 Northfield Road, King's Norton, Birmingham B30 1JH, England. Telephone: 0121 433 3727.

Idoloba – standardized Ginkgo supplement – is available from most good chemists and health food stores. In case of difficulty telephone 01932 336366.

Manuka cold-pressed honey, Aloe Vera products, Linusit Gold Linseeds and extra virgin olive oil should all be available from wholefood outlets. Good health food stores are an excellent source of new food ideas and many of them will stock organic produce.

For stockist information on Manuka honey and Tea Tree Oil products, contact **New Zealand Natural Food Company**, Unit 7, 55–57 Park Royal Road, London NW10 7JP. Telephone: 0181 961 4410.

For more information about **Linusit Gold Linseeds,** contact **The Health and Diet Company,** Europa Park, Stoneclough Road, Radcliffe, Manchester M26 1GG. Telephone: 01204 707420.

For stockists of quality Aloe Vera products, write to **Xynergy Health Products,** Ash House, Stedham, Midhurst, West Sussex GU29 0PT. Telephone: 01730 813642.

AUSTRALIA

Blackmores, 23 Roseberry Street, Balgowlah 2093, New South Wales, Australia. Telephone: (02) 951 0111.
Hilton Lifestream, 3 Romsay Street, Waitara, NSW 2077. Telephone: (02) 487 1155.

NEW ZEALAND

Blackmores, 2 Parkhead Place, Albany, Auckland, New Zealand. Telephone: (09) 415 8585.

Red Seal Natural Health Ltd, 46 Honan Place, Avondale, Auckland. Telephone: (09) 828 0036.

TRANSCENDENTAL MEDITATION

For details of classes, books and tapes, Freephone UK 0800 269303 or 01695 51213.
Or write to **TM National Communications Office,** Beacon House, Willow Walk, Woodley Park, Skelmersdale, Lancashire WN8 6UR, enclosing a large s.a.e. Outside the UK, details should be in the telephone directory under TM or 'Transcendental Meditation'.

AUSTRALIA: Telephone: (03) 467 8911.
NEW ZEALAND: Telephone: (09) 522 1052.

WATER FILTER UNITS

Crystal Waymaster Kenwood, New Lane, Havant, Hampshire PO9 2NH. Telephone: 01705 476000.

NEW ZEALAND
Contamination Control Ltd, PO Box 14621, Auckland 6. Telephone: (09) 570 9135.

There are many companies worldwide providing effective water filter units. Look in your local Yellow Pages directory under 'Water Treatment & Equipment'.

Important reminder: Please do not write to any of

these organizations without enclosing international reply coupons or a stamped addressed envelope. If you are contacting a charity or non-profit making organization, ask if you can contribute to their expenses.

Important Note

Kathryn is always delighted to hear from readers and promises to read every letter but regrets that, due to the cost and time involved in dealing with a weekly avalanche of mail, she can no longer reply individually to everyone. She is unable to comment on specific cases unless accompanied by a doctor's letter of referral and a full medical/health history.

The information which Kathryn includes in her books, articles and lectures has been accumulated from her own personal research, training and experience which, from the feedback she has received, would appear to have helped many people. However, these guidelines are *not* intended to be prescriptive, nor are they an attempt to diagnose or treat any particular condition. If you are concerned *in any way* about your health, Kathryn recommends that you consult your own medical adviser without delay.

It is wise to keep your GP informed of the progress of any symptoms, of any dietary changes and of any supplement programme you decide to follow. Obtain as many details about your condition from your medical adviser as you can – and ask plenty of questions about any medicines which may be recommended – but do not stop taking any existing prescribed medication without first consulting your doctor.

Follow a sensible diet which contains a wide variety of fresh, unprocessed foods, take regular exercise and avoid cigarette smoke.

I hope that the words
which you've read in this book
have
created a spark somewhere,
fired your imagination,
raised a smile or two,
given you the incentive
to worry a little less,
to nurture yourself a little more
and remember that
Life is nothing without love and laughter.

Kathryn Marsden

Index

Main references are in **BOLD**